Lab Experiences for the Pharmacy Technician

Lab Experiences for the Pharmacy Technician

Mary E. Mohr, RPh, MS
Pharmacy Technician Program Director
Clarian Health Partners, Inc.
Methodist Campus
Indianapolis, Indiana

LIPPINCOTT WILLIAMS & WILKINS
A **Wolters Kluwer** Company

Philadelphia • Baltimore • New York • London
Buenos Aires • Hong Kong • Sydney • Tokyo

Acquisitions Editor: David B. Troy
Managing Editor: Matthew J. Hauber
Marketing Manager: Marisa A. O'Brien
Production Editor: Jennifer D. Glazer
Design Coordinator: Holly McLaughlin
Compositor: Circle Graphics

Copyright © 2006 Lippincott Williams & Wilkins

351 West Camden Street
Baltimore, MD 21201

530 Walnut Street
Philadelphia, PA 19106

Photographs in Chapters 6, 7, 8, 9, and 11 from Thompson JE. *A Practical Guide to Contemporary Pharmacy Practice.* 2nd Ed. Philadelphia: Lippincott Williams & Wilkins, 2004; all photos taken by Larry W. Davidow.

Photographs in Chapters 16 and 18 from Allen LV, Popovich NG, Ansel HC. *Ansel's Pharmaceutical Dosage Forms and Drug Delivery Systems.* 8th Ed. Philadelphia: Lippincott Williams & Wilkins, 2005.

Appendix prescriptions from Finkel R. *Patient Care Management Lab: A Workbook for Prescription Practice.* Philadelphia: Lippincott Williams & Wilkins, 2002.

Printed in China

Library of Congress Cataloging-in-Publication Data

Mohr, Mary E.
    Lab experiences for the pharmacy technician / Mary E. Mohr
        p. ; cm.
    ISBN-13: 978-0-7817-5665-5
    ISBN-10: 0-7817-5665-0
    1. Pharmacy technicians—Problems, exercises, etc.   I. Title.
    [DNLM: 1. Drug Compounding—Problems and Exercises. 2. Dosage Forms—Problems and Exercises. 3. Pharmaceutical Preparations—administration and dosage—Problems and Exercises. 4. Pharmacy—methods—Problems and Exercises.   QV 18.2 M699L 2006]
RS122.95.M64 2006
615'.19076—dc22

                                    2005025621

The publishers have made every effort to trace the copyright holders for borrowed material. If they have inadvertently overlooked any, they will be pleased to make the necessary arrangements at the first opportunity.

To purchase additional copies of this book, call our customer service department at **(800) 638-3030** or fax orders to **(301) 223-2320.** International customers should call **(301) 223-2300.**

Visit Lippincott Williams & Wilkins on the Internet: http://www.LWW.com. Lippincott Williams & Wilkins customer service representatives are available from 8:30 am to 6:00 pm, EST.

                                                    09 10
                                    5 6 7 8 9 10 11

This manual is dedicated to my family and friends who have supported me with their love and to all the students, past and present, who have inspired me with their quest for knowledge. This includes a special dedication to my granddaughters, Makayla and Amelia, who hold the promise of our future.

Preface

Lab Experiences for the Pharmacy Technician was designed for use by pharmacy technician students in a formal education program. This manual will provide the student with pre-lab preparation, step-by-step instructions for the hands-on portion of the learning experience, and follow-up questions to provoke reflection on the results of the lab so as to bring clarity to the work.

It is expected that the technician will have completed some core courses or be taking them concurrently. These courses would include medical terminology, pharmacy calculations, pharmacology for technicians, law and ethics, and a general pharmacy practice course.

The student should also have access to a reasonable complement of pharmacy reference books, including *Facts and Comparisons, Remington's Science and Practice of Pharmacy, Trissel's Handbook of Injectable Drugs, PDR for Nonprescription Drugs,* and *The Pediatric Dosage Handbook,* as well as a general pharmacy practice text for technicians.

▶ Organization of the Manual

Lab Experiences for the Pharmacy Technician is divided into three units: Unit I, Pharmacy Operations; Unit II, Extemporaneous Compounds; and Unit III, Intravenous Admixtures. Within the units, each chapter represents a complete laboratory lesson consisting of the following:

▶ **Objectives,** a list of competencies that should be attained during completion of the exercise.

▶ **Key Terms,** the basic vocabulary to be researched by the student prior to the lab for an understanding of the functions to be performed.

▶ **Equipment** and, in certain chapters, **Ingredients** needed for completion of the lab.

▶ **Pre-Lab Questions** covering background knowledge to be researched prior to completing the lab.

▶ **Lab Exercises** including, among other types of exercises, patient scenarios, prescription practice, and step-by-step exercises to help students acquire and demonstrate competencies in a laboratory setting before actual clinical experiences.

▶ **Post-Lab Analysis,** a series of questions designed for reflection to bring clarity to the lab exercise.

▶ Suggestions for Use

The intent of this manual is to encourage and develop in pharmacy technician students the critical thinking skills they will need to meet their responsibilities in the rapidly changing world of pharmacy. A thorough understanding of reference materials and their use is vitally important to the technician of the future. In the past, we felt that technicians performed only duties that did not require "professional judgment." It is now understood that technicians *must* have the "professional judgment" of a competent technician to prevent medication errors and the resulting litigation and must be cognizant of the decisions that require the "professional judgment" of a pharmacist.

The format and many of the exercises in *Lab Experiences for the Pharmacy Technician* are currently used in a lab course that includes two 2½-hour lab sessions each week. The students complete an entire chapter, including the pre- and post-lab questions, during the lab sessions. Generally, this requires that both of the lab sessions each week be devoted to completing one full chapter. Various reference books are available, and the instructor is available to answer questions. The students work individually and in small groups, requesting help only when they have exhausted their resources. The instructor assigns readings prior to lab, presents a short pre-lab lecture on the material, and provides a demonstration of new or unfamiliar procedures. The students' pre-lab work and calculations are checked before they begin, and pertinent questions may be asked to ascertain their understanding of the exercise. Students are reminded again that the instructor is always available to answer questions during the lab. As the students work at their own pace, the instructor performs random checks for proper technique and occasionally challenges a student with questions. After completion of the post-lab questions, the paperwork is left in the checking area (the pages are perforated for ease of removal) indicated by the instructor with the finished product. Completed and graded exercises may be stored in the folder on the inside back cover.

If the time frame is different for the laboratory work in your institution, the lab time can be shortened by having the student come to lab with the pre-lab questions completed. The post-lab questions could also be completed outside of lab time and turned in later. *Lab Experiences for the Pharmacy Technician* was designed to be used with any of the currently available pharmacy technician practice texts.

To provide additional practice for pharmacy technician students, an appendix of **Supplemental Prescriptions and Medication Orders** is included at the end of the text.

▶ Instructor Resources

For the instructor, *Lab Experiences for the Pharmacy Technician* is designed to provide an organization and approach for teaching pharmacy technician lab courses and to be an instrument for evaluating students' work. The lists of Equipment and Ingredients at the beginning of each chapter are provided as an aid to instructors preparing for a lab session. The appendix of Supplemental Prescriptions and Medication Orders can be used to give students additional prescription practice and augment the materials presented within each chapter.

In addition, an **Instructor's Resource CD-Rom** to accompany *Lab Experiences for the Pharmacy Technician* is available to faculty and includes the following:

▶ **Pharmacy Technician Dispensing Lab Simulator,** a realistic computer simulator that pharmacy technician lab students can use to practice entering patient prescription information in a lab setting. All of the drugs and sig codes used in the lab book are pre-entered into the simulator. A list of the drugs is included separately on the CD-ROM, as well as a list of the sig codes, which may be posted in the lab for students to reference.

▶ **Instructor's Guide,** including a complete answer key for each chapter, as well as tips for instructors.

▶ **PowerPoint Slide Presentations,** for use in facilitating the pre-lab lecture.

▶ **Final Lab Exams,** including both a Final Written Exam and a Final Lab Practical with Scoring Sheet.

▶ **Materials Needed to Teach a Dispensing Lab,** including a comprehensive List of Equipment and List of Chemicals needed and resources for purchasing both, as well as a complete list of Reference Books utilized.

Inquire through your local LWW sales representative or by contacting the publisher at educsales@lww.com.

Acknowledgments

The preparation of this manual has been an adventure facilitated by a number of people. The assistance of the very professional publishing staff at Lippincott Williams & Wilkins is greatly appreciated. The constant advice and support of David Troy and Matt Hauber were invaluable. My thanks to the reviewers, named below, for their insights and advice, which provided expert guidance to this publication. Thanks also to Thomas Mohr, DO, and the residents and staff of the Michigan State Adult Medicine Clinic for providing handwritten prescriptions and to Michael Mohr, DO, for the handwritten Medication Orders.

Reviewers

James Austin
Texas Christian University
Weatherford, Texas

Edgar Cortes
Salt Lake/Tooele Applied Technology
   College
Salt Lake City, Utah

George Fakhoury, MD, DORCP, CMA
Silicon Valley College
Walnut Creek, California

Sara Love, CPhT
Apollo College
Portland, Oregon

Michael Parker, CPhT, EMT
Kaiser Permanente
Falls Church, Virginia

Debra L. Peelor
Bidwell Training Center
Pittsburgh, Pennsylvania

Anne E. Redmond, CPhT
Baker College
Flint, Michigan

Douglas Scribner, CPhT
Albuquerque TVI Community College
Albuquerque, New Mexico

Christina Seeger, CPhT
Apollo College
Portland, Oregon

Ray Vellenga, MS
Century College
White Bear Lake, Minnesota

Mark Williams
Mercy College of Northwest Ohio
Toledo, Ohio

Mahnaz Younes Abhari, PharmD
Northern Virginia Community College
Annandale, Virginia

Contents

Pharmacy Operations

CHAPTER 1

Communicating with Patients and Healthcare Professionals

TERMS

Patient profile
Controlled substances
DEA number
DAW
Stat
HIPAA

EQUIPMENT

Pharmacy reference books
Communication text
Pharmacy practice text

OBJECTIVES

▶ Evaluate an outpatient prescription for completeness.

▶ Develop the proper technique for gathering needed information from the patients and healthcare professionals.

▶ Demonstrate the ability to defuse difficult situations with anxious and upset patients and healthcare professionals

▶ List ways to accommodate special-needs patients.

▶ Assess the urgency of orders and prioritize work.

Effective communication skills enhance the professionalism of the technician, creating a feeling of trust and mutual respect with patients and other healthcare professionals. Appropriate interview techniques will put the patient at ease as they are asked for personal health information. Answer the following questions in preparation for the laboratory exercise.

▶ Pre-Lab Questions

1. List the information that must be on each prescription.

   _____

   _____

   _____

2. If the strength of a multiple-strength drug is omitted from the prescription, describe the action you would take as a technician.

   _____

   _____

   _____

3. The patient does not speak English and you speak only English. What are some possible ways to gather needed information?

   _____

   _____

   _____

4. When preparing prescriptions for a patient with limited vision, what are some things you can do to help differentiate between his medications?

   _____

   _____

   _____

5. Describe ways to communicate with a patient who is hearing impaired.

   _____

   _____

6. Discuss some methods for communicating with angry or upset patients or health-care professionals to defuse the situation.

_____

_____

_____

7. List rules for refilling prescriptions for controlled substances.

_____

_____

▶ Lab Exercises

Patient Scenarios

With a partner, act out the following scenarios. Take turns being the technician. Use the checklist following the scenarios to evaluate your partner's patient interviewing skills. Discuss the responses of the technician in the scenario with your partner and list other responses that may be more or less appropriate.

Scenario 1

Technician: "Hello, Mrs. Smith. How are you today?"

Mrs. Smith: "Well, it's raining so my arthritis is terrible. Every joint in my body aches. The doctor keeps giving me more medicine, but nothing helps. I don't know why I bother coming here."

Technician: "I'm sorry you're not feeling well, Mrs. Smith. Could I have your address and phone number so I can locate your file in the computer?"

Mrs. Smith: "As long as I've been coming here you should have all that by now. I'm going to call a cab so I can get home."

Technician: "Of course we have all your information in the computer, Mrs. Smith, but I just need a number to verify that I have the correct file. Do you have your patient ID card?"

Mrs. Smith: "Oh, here it is. Now how soon can you fill these six prescriptions? I'm calling a cab, and it will be here in 15 minutes. Surely it won't take longer than 15 minutes."

Technician: "Before you call the cab, I have a few questions. Do you have any drug allergies besides the codeine we have listed in the computer?"

Mrs. Smith: "I've already told you my allergies. Why do you keep asking me that? Oh, by the way, I did develop a rash when I took that new antibiotic last week."

Technician: "Okay, Mrs. Smith, I'll make a note of that for the pharmacist. Would you like to pick up your prescriptions later so you can go home now, or did you want to wait for them?"

Mrs. Smith: "Neither. I want them to be ready when the cab gets here, and would you also fill my old arthritis prescription. Maybe if I take it with the new one, I'll finally get some relief."

Technician: "Mrs. Smith, the pharmacist may want to discuss the new arthritis medicine with you when your order is ready. There are several people ahead of you, so it will be 20 to 30 minutes. Let the cab driver know that, and then have a seat."

Scenario 2

Technician: "Pharmacy, this is John, the technician, speaking."

Nurse: "Well, John, this is Marge. I am the nurse on 3B who ordered a stat medication for my very ill patient over a half hour ago. Do you understand what the word stat means?"

Technician: "If you will give me the information again, I will check on your order immediately and send it up to you."

Nurse: "I told you, I ordered the med over a half hour ago. Now stop wasting time, and bring it up to 3B now!!"

Technician: "Would you please give me the name of the patient again?"

Nurse: "Are you a bunch of idiots down there? We are incredibly busy up here with very ill patients, and you guys in pharmacy can't even fill a simple stat order."

Technician: "Look, Marge, I'm really sorry your order didn't arrive on time. If you'll trust me with the information, I will personally find the order, have it checked by a pharmacist, and deliver it to you."

Nurse: "It's been a really hectic day, John. I'm sorry I took my frustration out on you. If you could just get an ampule of Lasix 40 mg for Samuel Schmidt on 3B, I can take care of my patient. I know the pharmacist on the floor verified the order and entered it in the computer."

Technician: "I'll have the Lasix in your hand in 15 minutes."

Scenario 3

Mrs. Mendez arrives at the pharmacy with her empty Xanax prescription vial on April 4th. She speaks very little English but has brought her teenage daughter to interpret for her. When you enter the prescription number into the computer, you discover that, although she has used only two of the five refills authorized, the prescription was written in August of last year. With your partner, develop an appropriate dialog with the patient and/or her daughter. Keep in mind the HIPAA regulations on confidentiality in determining whether you may speak to her daughter about her mother's prescription. What other communication options might be available to aid in this scenario?

Checklist for Technician Interviewing Skills

Technician Name _____   Evaluator _____

	Greets patient or healthcare professional appropriately
	Asks content questions to clarify and complete required information
	Speaks in a clear and understandable manner at appropriate level
	Accepts responses and gives positive reinforcement
	Establishes rapport and demonstrates empathy both verbally and with body language
	Answers patient concerns or makes notes to refer the patient to the pharmacist

Checklist for Technician Interviewing Skills

Technician Name _____   Evaluator _____

	Greets patient or healthcare professional appropriately
	Asks content questions to clarify and complete required information
	Speaks in a clear and understandable manner at appropriate level
	Accepts responses and gives positive reinforcement
	Establishes rapport and demonstrates empathy both verbally and with body language
	Answers patient concerns or makes notes to refer the patient to the pharmacist

Prescription Practice

Examine the following prescriptions for completeness. In the blanks next to each prescription, note any missing or questionable information, and determine whether the information can be obtained from the patient or will require a call to the physician. Then proceed to the next exercise.

PRESCRIPTION 1.1

John Koth, MD
Phone: 783-4068
1802 North Andrews, Minneapolis, MN

Name: Adrian Skinner 120 Sand, Minneapolis

RX: AMOXICILLIN
       # 30

Sig: 1 CAP TID x 10 d

                                    John Koth, M.D.
———————————————   —————————————
Dispense as written   May substitute

_____
_____
_____
_____
_____

PRESCRIPTION 1.2

James Jones, DO
Phone: 261-9438

Name: Janie Simmons

RX: Vasotec 10mg

Dispense: #30

Sig: 1 tab qd a.m.

                                    James Jones, D.O.
———————————————   —————————————
Dispense as written   May substitute

_____
_____
_____
_____
_____

Patient Interviews

Using the patient profile charts that follow, conduct patient interviews to prepare to fill the prescriptions. Use this exercise to develop interview skills prior to data entry in a software program. Keep in mind the proper technique for patient interviews. Include questions about allergies, herbal and over the counter medicines used, and prescriptions filled at another pharmacy. Continue to work with your assigned partner taking turns being the patient and the technician. As the patient, be creative with your responses. As the technician, respond appropriately to the information received from the patient. Be concise in documenting information and use appropriate terminology. Do not enter derogatory comments about the patient in the comments section!

Patient	Address	Phone	D.O.B.	Allergies	Cash/Ins	Comments
Adrian Skinner						

Rx #	Drug	Quantity	Date	Directions	Prescriber	Pharmacy comments

Patient	Address	Phone	D.O.B.	Allergies	Cash/Ins	Comments
Janie Simmons						

Rx #	Drug	Quantity	Date	Directions	Prescriber	Pharmacy comments

▶ Post-Lab Analysis

1. On a very busy day in the pharmacy, the following patients have arrived with prescriptions. If they arrived in the following order, indicate by numbering, the order in which they might be filled.

    _____   Mrs. Jones has six refill bottles.

    _____   Mr. Smith has just seen the doctor for his yearly check-up and has five new prescriptions for his maintenance medications.

    _____   Mrs. Angelo has brought her ill child to see the doctor and has prescriptions for an antibiotic and an otic solution. The baby is crying.

    _____   Jane Saver has arrived from the dental clinic where two teeth were extracted. She has a prescription for a pain killer, and blood drips on the counter as she stumbles to find a seat.

2. Give the rationale for the order in which you prioritized the prescriptions. Include the dialog you would have with each patient to give them an approximate wait time.

    Mrs. Jones   _____

    _____

    _____

    Mr. Smith   _____

    _____

    _____

    Mrs. Angelo _____

    _____

    _____

    Jane Saver   _____

    _____

    _____

    _____

Data Entry of Prescriptions

OBJECTIVES

▶ List the various interactions encountered during data entry of prescriptions.

▶ Demonstrate appropriate actions when computer software indicates an interaction.

▶ Describe procedures for attaining refill authorization when required.

▶ Discuss steps involved in transfer of prescription to another pharmacy.

▶ List basic procedures for third-party billing.

Accurate data entry is vitally important to prevent medication errors and drug interactions and to assure correct reimbursement from third-party payors. The questions on drug interactions will aid in understanding the necessity of the patient profile, including diagnosis, allergies, and current medications, both OTC and prescription. Permission to override an interaction warning must come from the supervising pharmacist. With a basic knowledge of third-party insurance plans and the terminology involved, the technician can become skillful in on-line adjudication, allowing the pharmacist more time for improved pharmaceutical care of patients.

▶ Pre-Lab Questions

1. Discuss the significance rating for drug-drug and drug-food interactions as described in the Drug Interaction Facts.

   _____

   _____

   _____

2. Differentiate the meanings of major, moderate, and minor severity of a drug-drug or drug-food interaction.

   _____

   _____

   _____

3. When entering prescriptions for an asthmatic patient for albuterol, salmeterol, and fluticasone inhalers, the software indicates a duplicate therapy interaction. Discuss the reasons for this and possible rationale for overriding this message.

   _____

   _____

   _____

4. Most HMO's have a contract with the participating pharmacies that states a monthly capitation fee for each patient. This means that the pharmacy gets paid the same amount every month for each patient member of that plan regardless of the number or cost of prescriptions required by that member. Two patients belong to the same HMO where the monthly capitation fee is $100 (the insurance company will pay the pharmacy $100 each month for that patient), and the patient has a $5.00 dollar co-pay to the pharmacy for each prescription.

   Mr. Jones has three monthly prescriptions costing $26, $43, and $38. Mr. Allen has two prescriptions costing $120 and $18. What was the pharmacy's profit or loss for each patient? What was the total profit or loss for the two patients? Do the math calculations in the space on the next page.

Mr. Jones monthly prescription cost _____ Mr. Jones capitation fee + co-pays _____

Pharmacy profit or loss from Mr. Jones prescriptions _____

Mr. Allen's monthly prescription cost _____ Mr. Allen's capitation fee + co-pays _____

Pharmacy profit or loss from Mr. Allen's prescription_____

Combined profit or loss from both patients _____

Discuss the risk involved with reimbursement based on a capitation fee.

_____

_____

_____

5. Mrs. James' insurance company reimburses the pharmacy using the formula AWP minus 10% plus a $5.00 dispensing fee. Mrs. James pays a $10.00 co-pay for each prescription. The actual acquisition cost of her medicine is $98.00 for 100 tablets, and the AWP is $120 for 100 tablets. What will the pharmacy receive from the insurance company for a 30-day supply if she takes one tablet bid? How much gross profit will the pharmacy receive for each prescription? Perform the calculations below. Label your answers.

Acquisition cost for 60 tablets_____58.8_____(a) AWP for 60 tablets_____72_____(b)

Insurance reimbursement for 60 tablets (AWP −10%) _____ + $5.00 dispensing fee___69.8___(c)

Insurance reimbursement (c)_____ + co-pay_____−acquisition cost (a)_____ = _____
     gross profit

6. Marcia Shaver returns to the pharmacy after 30 days requesting a refill on her Advair Diskus. The physician has not authorized any refills. List several ways a technician could obtain refill authorization.

_____

_____

_____

7. Mrs. Bayfield has moved from an area near your pharmacy to a new home across town. The pharmacy technician in the new pharmacy she has chosen calls to transfer her prescriptions. List the required information that could be transferred between the two technicians and the information that must be conveyed between the two pharmacists.

_____

_____

_____

_____

8. Susan Smiley brings in a prescription for her granddaughter, Shelley, who is visiting for a few weeks during the summer. The antibiotic prescribed for Shelley is very expensive, and Susan asks you to fill the prescription with her name and submit it to her husband's insurance company. What would your response by and why?

_____

_____

_____

_____

▶ Lab Exercises

As you work through the lab exercises in this chapter, use the following Patient Profile Charts to practice gathering and recording pertinent patient information for "Susan Smiley" and "Marcia Shaver" from the prescriptions and insurance cards that follow. Pair with another student to practice the patient-technician interaction when a new prescription is presented to the pharmacy. Include the insurance information from their insurance cards. Using a computer software program, enter the prescriptions for the patients, and print the labels and paperwork. These should be turned in for grading before the next exercise when the prescriptions will be filled and labeled. Save the labels and paperwork to be used for the Chapter 3 Lab Exercise.

Patient Profile Charts

Patient	Address	Phone	D.O.B.	Allergies	Cash/Ins	Comments
					Co-Pay	Plan #
						ID #

Rx #	Drug	Quantity	Date	Directions	Prescriber	Pharmacy comments

Patient	Address	Phone	D.O.B.	Allergies	Cash/Ins	Comments
					Co-Pay	Plan #
						ID #

Rx #	Drug	Quantity	Date	Directions	Prescriber	Pharmacy comments

Prescription Practice

Assess the following prescriptions for accuracy and completeness and check for reasonable dosage and drug interactions. In the blanks next to each prescription, note any action needed. When complete, update the patient profile, including any third-party information, and enter the prescriptions in the computer.

PRESCRIPTION 2.1

Joseph Manakee, MD
1820 South Street, Hale, AL 40301

Name: Susan Smiley   64 Macon Road, Hale, AL

RX: Pencillin 500mg

Disp: #28

Sig: 1 tab P.O qid

Refill 1 2 3 NR

_____   *Joseph Manakee, MD*
Dispense as written   May substitute

_____

_____

_____

_____

_____

PRESCRIPTION 2.2

Joseph Manakee, MD
1820 South Street, Hale, AL 40301

Name: Susan Smiley   64 Macon Road, Hale, AL

RX: Ortho-Novum 1/35-28

Disp: # 6 mon

Sig: 1 tab PO qd

Refill 1 2 3 NR

_____   *Joseph Manakee, MD*
Dispense as written   May substitute

_____

_____

_____

_____

PRESCRIPTION 2.3

Joseph Manakee, MD
1820 South Street, Hale, AL 40301

Name: Susan Smiley   64 Macon Road, Hale, AL

RX: Tylnol codeine #3

Disp: #20

Sig: 1-2 PO qid prn pain

Refill 1 2 3 NR

_____   *Joseph Manakee, MD*
Dispense as written   May substitute

_____
_____
_____
_____
_____

PRESCRIPTION 2.4

Thomas Moore, DO
5403 Half Moon, Lansing, MI

Name: Alaine Smithers   2201 Nation St, Ann Arbor, MI

RX: VICODIN

Disp: #60

Sig: 1-2 po q4-6h prn pain

Refill 1 2 3 NR

_____   *T. Moore, DO*
Dispense as written   May substitute

_____
_____
_____
_____
_____

PRESCRIPTION 2.5

Thomas Moore, DO
5403 Half Moon, Lansing, MI

Name: Alaine Smithers   2201 Nation St, Ann Arbor, MI

RX: ACETAMINOPHEN 500 mg

Disp: #100

Sig: 1-2 prn break through pain

Refill 1 2 3 NR

_____   *T. Moore, DO*
Dispense as written   May substitute

_____
_____
_____
_____
_____

PRESCRIPTION 2.6

Thomas Moore, DO
5403 Half Moon, Lansing, MI

Name: Alaine Smithers   2201 Nation St, Ann Arbor, MI

RX: SKELAXIN 400 mg.

Disp: #60

Sig: 2t PO tid X₁₀ d prn back spasm

Refill 1 2 3 NR

_____   T. Moore, DO
Dispense as written   May substitute

PRESCRIPTION 2.7

Ann Hennessey, MD
1214 Pine Lane, Cold River, VT 60503

Name: Marcia M. Shaver   1203 Grant, Cold River, VT

RX: Serevent inhaler

Disp: #1

Sig: 1 inhl prn asthma attack

Refill 1 2 3 NR

_____   Ann Hennessey, MD
Dispense as written   May substitute

PRESCRIPTION 2.8

Ann Hennessey, MD
1214 Pine Lane, Cold River, VT 60503

Name: Marcia M. Shaver   1203 Grant, Cold River, VT

RX Albuterol Inhaler

Disp #1

Sig 1 inhl bid for asthma

Refill 1 2 3 NR

_____   Ann Hennessey, MD
Dispense as written   May substitute

PRESCRIPTION 2.9

Ann Hennessey, MD
1214 Pine Lane, Cold River, VT 60503

Name: Marcia M. Shaver   1203 Grant, Cold River, VT

RX: Advair Diskus

Disp: #1

Sig: 2 puffs bid for Asthma

Refill 1 2 3 NR

_____   *Ann Hennessey, MD*
Dispense as written   May substitute

_____

_____

_____

_____

_____

Third Party Insurance

The following insurance cards were presented by the indicated patients. Enter the required information in the appropriate patient profiles. Turn the profile page in to document your work and then enter the information in a computer software system and print the prescription paperwork and labels.

K-Plan HMO	**Group:** 0000007259
	Member # 0000653478
	Effective: 01/01/05

Membr: Marcia M. Shaver
PCP: Ann Hennessey, MD
Phone #: 654-831-0457
Network: Kaptan Medical Group

Co-pays: RX: Generic $10, Select $30, Non-Select 50% of the cost with a $50 minimum

_____

_____

_____

_____

Axiom Insurance		**PPO**
Member Name:	Axiom Rx Network	
Susan Smiley	Office Call	20%
	Urgent Care	20%
Subscriber Name:	Rx	20%/10%
John Smiley	Inpatient	20%
	Outpatient	20%
Identification Number:		
YTN413258066		
Group No.: 0060412		
Plan No.: 465		
Beginning Date: 01/01/05		

_____

_____

_____

_____

▶ Post-Lab Analysis

1. Discuss any drug-drug or drug-food interaction(s) that would be a concern with Susan Smiley's prescriptions. Include the type of interaction, the significance rating, the severity of the interaction(s), and the need to involve the pharmacist.

    _____

    _____

    _____

2. As a technician, with knowledge of a possible interaction, how would you express the offer of counseling by the pharmacist? What advice would you expect the pharmacist to give the patient to manage the possible interaction(s)?

    _____

    _____

    _____

    _____

3. Name the type of interaction indicated by the software after entering the three prescriptions for Marcia Shaver? Tell why the pharmacist would not override this interaction.

    _____

    _____

    _____

4. Are the directions for use consistent with your knowledge of Marcia Shaver's three inhalers? Discuss why a call to the physician might be necessary.

    _____

    _____

    _____

5. Alaine Smithers has sustained a painful back injury. The doctor is trying to provide ample pain relief with minimal usage of controlled drugs. What problem might result from using acetaminophen in addition to Vicodin?

    _____

    _____

6. What might the pharmacist recommend to Alaine Smithers' physician to provide adequate pain relief without risk of toxicity?

_____

_____

7. Alaine Smithers' insurance company replies during on-line adjudication that Skelaxin is a drug that requires prior authorization. What steps might be taken to resolve this situation?

_____

_____

_____

_____

8. If the AWP of Susan Smiley's prescriptions were $7.50, $21.00, and $5.00, what would her co-pay total be if all three were filled with generics?

_____

9. K-Plan classifies Serevent as a Select drug and Advair as a Non-Select drug. If the albuterol were filled generically and the physician discontinued the Serevent, what amount would you charge Marcia for her two prescriptions?

_____

10. If Dr. Hennessey was not Marcia's established Primary Care Provider, how would that affect the cost of her prescriptions? Why?

_____

CHAPTER 3

Filling and Labeling the Prescription

TERMS

Labeling
Red C stamp
Expiration dating
Auxiliary labels
Beyond use date
mg/kg
BSA
Clark's Rule
Young's Rule
Fried's Rule
Drug-specific pediatric doses
Black box warning
Chemical name
NDC number

EQUIPMENT

Pharmacy reference books:
   a. *Facts and Comparisons*
   b. *Pediatric Dosing Handbook*
Pharmacy software
Prescription vials
Counting tray/spatula
Package inserts
Medications or placebo
Alcohol for cleaning counters
Alcohol wipes for cleaning trays
Pharmacy tweezers
Prescription label tape

OBJECTIVES

▶ Demonstrate labeling for an outpatient prescription.

▶ Correctly file prescriptions for controlled and noncontrolled drugs.

▶ Compare the label with the hard copy of the prescription to ensure accuracy.

▶ Check the appropriateness of the dose and dosage form for the patient.

▶ Procure the correct medication from the shelf and check the expiration date.

▶ Choose the proper size and type of container needed for the medication.

▶ Count or measure the medication, place in container, and affix label.

▶ Place the prescription and paperwork in an organized manner for the pharmacist to perform the final check.

This chapter combines the knowledge from the first and second chapters with the ability to complete the processing of the prescription and prepare the materials for the final check by the pharmacist. Calculations of pediatric doses using four different formulas provides a basis for comparing the formula results with the manufacturer-specific dosing guidelines found in the package insert. Research the following questions in preparation for the Laboratory Exercises.

▶ Pre-Lab Questions

1. Discuss the various filing systems for prescriptions and when stamping a Red C would be required on a prescription (if applicable in your state).

   _____

   _____

   _____

2. Would it be safe to dispense a medication that expires December of 2004 on November 15, 2004 if the prescription reads dispense 60 capsules with directions to take one capsule two times a day? Discuss the rationale for your answer.

   _____

   _____

   _____

3. When dispensing a prescription for Cipro, what auxiliary labels should be attached to the vial?

   _____

   _____

   _____

4. Makayla Mayer, a 6-year-old female patient, weighs 50 pounds and is 45 inches tall. She has otitis media, and although allergic to penicillin, she has been able to tolerate cephalexin. The usual adult dose of cephalexin is 250 mg q6h. Calculate the correct pediatric dose using Young's Rule, Clark's Rule, and BSA (assume 1.73 m^2 is average adult BSA). Then calculate the dose using drug-specific information from the package insert (25–50 mg/kg/d in four divided doses). Label each answer clearly.

5. Compare and discuss the results of Makayla Mayer's dose calculations.

   _____

   _____

   _____

6. Tyler Zen is an 8-week-old male infant weighing 14 pounds. The doctor wants to prescribe captopril for him. The usual adult starting dose is 25 mg. The drug-specific dosing information for an infant from the reference material is 0.01 mg/kg. Calculate the dose using Fried's Rule, Clark's Rule, and the drug-specific information. Be sure to circle and clearly mark each answer.

7. Compare and discuss the results of Tyler Zen's dosing calculations.

   _____

   _____

   _____

8. Based on your experience with the previous dosing calculation exercises, what is the most accurate method for determining the appropriate pediatric dose if the information is available?

   _____

9. When filling a prescription for a patient who's profile indicates renal impairment, how would you determine if it would create a problem with the prescribed drug?

   _____

   _____

▶ Lab Exercises

Reading Package Inserts

Using the Package Insert Worksheets on the following pages and two different package inserts available in the lab, find and record the requested information. The package insert is a valuable source of information that is readily available when filling prescriptions. Develop a proficiency in locating information in the insert.

Package Insert Worksheet

Drug Brand Name _____

Generic Name _____

Chemical Name _____

NDC Number _____

Dosage Forms Available _____

Usual Dose Range _____

Indication (s) _____

Contraindications _____

_____

Pregnancy Category _____

Route of Elimination _____

Adverse Effects _____

_____

Summarize Black Box Warning (if any) _____

_____

_____

_____

Package Insert Worksheet

Drug Brand Name _____

Generic Name _____

Chemical Name _____

NDC Number _____

Dosage Forms Available _____

Usual Dose Range _____

Indication (s) _____

Contraindications _____

_____

Pregnancy Category _____

Route of Elimination _____

Adverse Effects _____

_____

Summarize Black Box Warning (if any) _____

_____

_____

_____

Prescription Filling

Using the labels created from the corrected prescriptions in Chapter 2, begin the process of filling and labeling prescriptions.

Steps:

1. Separate the paperwork according to patient.
2. Begin filling the prescriptions for one patient.
3. Double-check each label with the hard copy of the prescription.
4. Re-check the patient profile to address any concerns, including whether the patient has requested non–child proof caps or has a disability that may require special handling.
5. Procure the medication for the first prescription from the shelf.
6. Check the expiration date on the bottle as you retrieve it from the shelf.
7. Verify the drug name and strength of the medication with the hard copy and the label.
8. Using the spatula and counting tray, count the number of doses (if applicable).
9. Using the measuring guideline on the counting tray as a guide, select the appropriate size container and pour the medication into the vial.
10. Re-check the drug name and strength on the prescription label, the hard copy of the prescription, and the medication bottle as you pour the medication into the container.
11. Apply the label to the container, add the necessary auxiliary labels, and perform another check as you assemble the paperwork and containers in an organized manner for the final check by the pharmacist.

> Watch for look-alike and sound-alike drugs!

> Read label three times

> Keep each patient's prescriptions together

12. Repeat these steps for each prescription until they become routine, developing optimal speed and accuracy.

▶ Post-Lab Analysis

1. Which of Susan Smiley's prescriptions requires that a patient package insert be included with each prescription?

   _____

2. What does the #3 in the Tylenol with Codeine prescription indicate?

   _____

3. Which two auxiliary labels would need to be attached to the prescription vials containing the Tylenol with Codeine and the Vicodin?

_____

_____

4. If Susan Smiley requested a generic for her oral contraceptive prescription, what reference book would give the bioequivalence rating of the generic carried by your pharmacy?

_____

_____

5. Alaine Smithers has arthritis and has requested non–child proof caps on her prescriptions. What documentation would you place on the prescription for future reference?

_____

_____

6. After phoning Dr. Moore's office to obtain his DEA number for the Vicodin prescription and receiving the following number, perform a check to see if this is a valid DEA: BM2398320.

Describe what action you would take if it were an invalid number

_____

_____

7. After a phone call to Dr. Hennessey, the Serevent Diskus was discontinued because salmeterol is included in Advair. Describe the difference between the _administration_ of albuterol in a metered dose inhaler and the Advair in the Diskus formulation.

_____

_____

_____

_____

8. Would either the albuterol MDI or the Advair Diskus require a shake well label? Why or why not?

_____

_____

_____

9. If the doctor indicated that Marcia should use a spacer, which of the two devices would it be used with? Describe the use of a spacer and the advantages to the patient.

_____

_____

_____

10. You receive a prescription for Benadryl elixir, 1 bottle, with directions for the patient to take 5 ml tid. You have only the generic available in a 4-ounce bottle. What is the generic name that you will put on the label?

_____

How many doses will the patient receive if you dispense the whole bottle? _____

How many days will the bottle last? _____

What size oral syringe would you give the patient? _____

Nonprescription Drugs

OBJECTIVES

◗ Develop a working knowledge of over-the-counter (OTC) drug products and their uses.

◗ List products that are sugar-free and those that are alcohol-free.

◗ Discuss the risk of exceeding the maximum daily dose of acetaminophen when using OTC products in addition to prescription products.

◗ Demonstrate technician initiatives when OTC purchases contain ingredients that may interact with a patient's prescription medications.

◗ Demonstrate the technician's role in the sale of OTC-exempt narcotics.

◗ Differentiate between water-soluble and fat-soluble vitamins.

▶ Pre-Lab Questions

1. Define an analgesic and give examples of OTC analgesics.

   _____

   _____

2. List three common OTC antihistamines, and describe their uses and side effects.

   _____

   _____

   _____

3. Explain the difference in side effects that may be expected when changing from Benadryl to Claritin.

   _____

   _____

   _____

4. Compare and contrast the therapeutic actions of NSAIDS, acetaminophen, and aspirin considering antipyretic, anti-inflammatory, and analgesic effects.

   _____

   _____

   _____

5. Describe the procedure for selling exempt (schedule V) narcotics that do not require a prescription.

   _____

   _____

   _____

6. Which OTC H-2 antagonist causes the most drug interactions?

   _____

7. Why would a proton pump inhibitor (PPI), such as Prilosec, not be effective in relieving heartburn?

   _____

   _____

CHAPTER 4 Nonprescription Drugs   **33**

8. Compare and contrast the three types of laxatives: fiber, stimulant, and stool softener.

_____

_____

_____

9. Name three different ways that antifungals are formulated for topical administration.

_____

_____

10. What is the maximum daily dose of acetaminophen? What is the major risk of exceeding this dose and/or combining acetaminophen with alcohol consumption?

_____

_____

11. List three sugar-free liquid cold preparations. Describe patients for whom sugar content is a concern.

_____

_____

_____

12. List one cold preparation that contains alcohol and three that are alcohol-free. Describe patients for whom alcohol content is a concern.

_____

_____

_____

13. List the fat-soluble vitamins. Describe the reason patients need to be especially careful not to overdose on these vitamins.

_____

_____

_____

▶ Lab Exercises

Patient Scenarios

Often OTC purchases occur when the pharmacist has already performed counseling or after counseling has been refused by the patient. An alert and knowledgeable technician will take the initiative to involve the pharmacist and avert an adverse reaction. Note your concerns with the following patient scenarios. Choose a partner and practice appropriate dialog between the technician and patient and the technician and the pharmacist.

Scenario 1

Mr. Jones arrives at the pharmacy counter to pick up his prescription for Vicodin. Since he called the refill line earlier, it is ready for him. He has brought a large bottle of extra strength Tylenol to purchase along with his prescription. You remember typing the directions for the Vicodin as 1 to 2 tablets every 3 to 4 hours. Discuss the action you would take and your conversation with the patient and/or the pharmacist.

_____

_____

_____

_____

_____

Scenario 2

Sally Smith asks you to add a large bottle of Nyquil to her order as she picks up her refills. She says she has had a hacking cough that keeps her awake at night. You note as you bring her prescription bag to the counter that she is taking glucophage, insulin, and enalapril. Why would you take the initiative to involve the pharmacist in this transaction? What could be the cause of her cough?

_____

_____

_____

Scenario 3

Joan Kennedy arrives at the pharmacy counter to pick up her prescription refill for the Plavix she has been taking since her recent heart attack. She asks you to also ring up her OTC purchase of Arthritis Strength Bufferin as she has been experiencing some morning stiffness in her hands. Why would you want to involve the pharmacist in this transaction?

_____

_____

_____

Scenario 4

Chris Keller refuses counseling from the pharmacist as he picks up his prescription for Cipro. He says he has taken it before and knows all about it. As you ring up the OTC items he wants to purchase, you notice a large bottle of Tums. He tells you that the Cipro caused him to have an unsettled stomach the last time he took it, so he wants to take a Tums with each dose. How would you involve the pharmacist without upsetting the patient?

_____

_____

_____

Scenario 5

Mrs. Peron is in a hurry to pick up her refill for Ditropan XL, but she asks you to ring up her OTC purchase of Benadryl since she has been bothered by some seasonal allergies. What concern would you have that might prompt you to involve the pharmacist in this transaction?

_____

_____

_____

Drug Familiarization

Using reference books, the OTC drug section in your lab, or a trip to the nearest pharmacy, fill in the blank spaces in the following chart to use as a personal reference. Familiarize yourself with the ingredients of the more common OTC preparations and their uses. This will prepare you to aid the pharmacist in providing good pharmaceutical care.

Category	Brand Name	Active Ingredients	Use
Analgesic/antipyretic		Acetaminophen	
(salicylate)	Bayer aspirin		
(NSAID)	Motrin IB		
	Aleve		
Pediatric analgesic/ antipyretic formulations	Tylenol drops Tylenol liquid Motrin suspension Motrin drops	Acetaminophen 80 mg/0.8 ml Acetaminophen 80 mg/1/2 tsp Ibuprofen 100 mg/5 ml Ibuprofen 50 mg/1.25 ml	
Antacid liquid/tablets	Maalox		
	Mylanta		

Category	Brand Name	Active Ingredients	Use
	Gaviscon		
	Tums		
	Pepto Bismol		
H-2 Antagonists	Zantac 75		
	Pepcid AC		
	Pepcid Complete		
	Tagamet HB		
Antidiarrheals	Kaopectate		
	Imodium AD		
	Donnagel		
	Pepto Bismol		
Fiber laxative	Metamucil		

Category	Brand Name	Active Ingredients	Use
Stimulant laxative	Dulcolax	Bisacodyl	
Anti-gas	Mylicon		
Stool softener	Colace		
	Surfak		
Hemorrhoidal preparation	Preparation H		
	Anusol		
	Anusol HC		
Vaginal antifungal	Monistat		
	Mycelex		
	Gyne-Lotrimin		
Topical antifungal	Tinactin		
	Micatin		

Category	Brand Name	Active Ingredients	Use
	Lotrimin A/F		
	Mycelex		
Topical antibiotics	Bacitracin		
	Neopsorin		
	Polysporin		
Topical steroid	Cortaid		
Vitamin A	Aquasol A Retinol	Fat soluble	
Vitamin B-1	thiamine	Water soluble	
Vitamin B-2	Riboflavin		
Vitamin B-3		Water soluble	
Vitamin	Pyridoxine	Water soluble	
Vitamin B-12			
Folic acid	Folate Folvite		
Vitamin C		Water soluble	
Vitamin____	ergocalciferol	Fat soluble	
Vitamin E	Alpha tocopheryl acetate		
Vitamin K	Menadiol		
Mineral: Iron (Fe)	Ferrous Sulfate 325 mg Ferro Sequels Ferrous Sulfate Elixir 220 mg/5 ml Fer In Sol drops 75 mg/0.6 ml	Equal 65 mg elemental iron 44 mg elemental iron 15 mg elemental iron/0.6 ml	

▶ Post-Lab Analysis

*Place a **P** in the space before the questions that require a pharmacist's intervention and a **T** in front of the questions that can be answered by the technician.*

1. _____ Mr. Jones wants to purchase a bottle of Maalox to replenish the family medicine cabinet. He asks if he should look in the aisle with the pain relievers (it relieves heartburn) or with the antacids.

2. _____ Susie Swover says her doctor told her to take one baby aspirin a day since her recent heart attack. She asks you what a "baby" aspirin is.

3. _____ Sally Smith brings a large bottle of extra strength acetaminophen to the counter. As you begin to process her purchase, she tells you she has a major headache and wants to get rid of it so she can go drinking with her friends. She says she's sure she'll need more acetaminophen tomorrow to help with the hangover.

4. _____ Christine Smith confides in you that she has just used a home pregnancy test and it was positive. She is purchasing a bottle of Nyquil to get rid of a "nasty cold" so she can get some sleep.

5. _____ Dr. James calls to see if your pharmacy carries a generic for Lotrimin cream in an OTC strength.

6. _____ Mike Malone asks you to recommend a cough syrup for him. He tells you that he is taking medication for asthma and blood pressure.

7. _____ Marcia Mack hands you a piece of paper with the word "diphenhydramine" written on it. She says her doctor told her to give this to her daughter for her allergies using the dosing directions on the bottle. Marcia wants you to help her find this medication.

8. _____ You answer the phone and the caller wants to know if bisacodyl and Dulcolax are the same thing.

9. _____ Mrs. Somers wants to know if the OTC Prilosec is the same strength as her prescription Prilosec.

10. _____ Sammy Southern wants you to recommend a laxative for him. You remember filling a prescription for Lomotil for him earlier in the week.

CHAPTER 5

Medication Orders–Inpatient

OBJECTIVES

▶ Demonstrate the ability to interpret medication orders using knowledge of medical terminology and abbreviations.

▶ Determine which entries on the medication order form are pertinent to the pharmacy.

▶ Accurately enter medication information to produce labels for cart fills.

▶ Demonstrate unit dose packaging.

▶ Fill patient-specific trays for medication carts.

▶ Demonstrate an understanding of automated dispensing systems.

TERMS

NKDA

Type 2 DM

Hyperlipidemia

IVNS

DX–diagnosis

PMHx–prior medical history

H/O–history of

C/O–complains of

Tob 1 ppd–tobacco 1 pack per day

Social ETOH–social alcohol drinker

0 illicits–no illicit drug use

SOAP–subjective-objective assessment plan

Unit dose

Pre-pack

Physician Order Entry

STAT order

PRN order

Automatic stop order

Medication automation systems

Pyxis Medstation

EQUIPMENT

Computer order entry system

Pharmacy reference books

Unit dose blister packs

Oral syringes

Drawers medication carts

Prescription vials

Small Ziploc® plastic bags

▶ Pre-Lab Questions

1. List the information that would be included on an inpatient medication form.

   _____

   _____

   _____

   _____

2. List information that would be required on an outpatient prescription form that would not be included on an inpatient medication form.

   _____

   _____

   _____

3. Explain the use of automatic stop orders, and identify several types of drugs often issued with automatic stop orders.

   _____

   _____

   _____

4. What is the usual time frame for a STAT order to be delivered to the floor?

   _____

5. List the types of professionals authorized to write prescription orders.

   _____

   _____

   _____

6. List the information required to be on the label of a drug pre-packed in unit dose packaging by pharmacy personnel.

   _____

   _____

   _____

7. What is used to determine the expiration date for medications pre-packed by the pharmacy?

_____

_____

8. What information needs to be on medications placed in an individual patient's drawer when using a manual-fill medication cart system?

_____

_____

9. What patient identification should be on the patient drawer in a medication cart?

_____

10. When using an automated dispensing system such as the Pyxis Medstation, why is it important to log out after each use?

_____

11. List some reasons why a discrepancy might be indicated by an automated dispensing system when the technician attempts to load a medication.

_____

_____

_____

12. Why is it important to report and document a discrepancy immediately when it is discovered?

_____

_____

_____

13. When multiple doses of a medication are loaded into one drawer and they have different expiration dates, how do you determine the expiration date that should be recorded for that drawer?

_____

_____

▶ Lab Exercises

Reading Medication Orders

Using your knowledge of medical terminology and available pharmacy reference books, interpret the following medical orders and progress notes for John Doe. Re-write the or-

Date/Time	Orders	Progress Notes

3/20/04 0700	Admit – Respiratory Unit
	
	Dx: Pneumonia
	   Asthma
	Condition: Fair
	V.S.: q4°
	Activity: BRP
	Nursing: Pulse Oximetry
	All: NKDA I&O, incentive
	   Spirometry
	Diet – Regular
	IVF: NS+20meq KCL
	   @ 125cc/hour
	O₂ NC 2-4 L/min
	   keep pulse ox >90%
	Rocephin 2gram IV q24°
	Zithromax 500mg p.o. day 1
	   then 250mg p.o. qd x 4 day
	Albuterol Nebulizer Treatment
	   q-2-4° PRN while awake
	Tylenol 500mg p.o. q8° PRN pain
	Ambien 10mg p.o. qHS/PRN insomnia
	MOM 15cc p.o. qd/PRN constipation
	Labs: CBC, 22, Bld cultures x2
	   CXR PA/LAT
		43 y/o ♂ c̄ H/o asthma presents c̄ ↑SOB/wheezing over past 3 days. Pt states he is coughing up rust-colored sputum and his fever has been as high as 102°
		
		PMHx: Asthma PSHx: hernia
		Meds: Albuterol NKDA
		   Advair 100/50
		Soc Hx: married – Lab Tech
		   ∅ Tob ∅ ETOH ∅ illicits
		FaHx: ♂ AKW ♀ Breast CA
		
		⊕ gen A/O moderate resp. distress
		V.S. T-101° P-88 R-20 130/82 pulse ox 90%
		CV – RRR
		Lung – Adequate BS coarse Rhonch LML
		   diffuse wheezes
		Abd Soft NT/ND +BS
		Ext – ∅ CCE
		A/P 1) Pneumonia
		   2) Asthma
		   Admit – Antibx – O₂
		   ✓ labs, CXR – Resp Treatment

MEDICAL ORDERS AND PROGRESS NOTES

EL-FR-NR-1001-1101

PATIENT INFORMATION

John Doe 43 y/o
8/29/60

CHART COPY

ders and progress notes on the blank lines below in layman's terms using no abbrevia-
tions. With a highlighter, indicate on the original form the lines that require an order to
be filled by the pharmacy.

_____

_____

_____

_____

_____

_____

_____

_____

_____

_____

_____

_____

_____

_____

_____

_____

Manual Cart Fills

With the increased technology available to pharmacies, manually filled medication carts
are being replaced by automated dispensing systems. However, there are still many small
hospitals and nursing homes where budget constraints necessitate the continued use of
manual-fill medication carts. Each pharmacy involved in manual cart fills will have poli-
cies for this procedure. This exercise is designed to present an overview of some basic
steps to accomplish this task. As with other tasks, it is important to learn the protocol of
the pharmacy setting in which you work.

Steps:

▶ The following patients are residents in a small nursing home that uses medication carts that are manually filled.

▶ Each drawer must be labeled with the patient's name, hospital number, and room number.

▶ The pharmacy exchanges the carts once a week, so each medication should contain a 7-day supply when returned to the nursing home.

▶ Some of the drawers may have unused doses left in them from the previous week. On the Medication List form, calculate the amount needed daily and the amount needed for 7 days.

▶ Then subtract the number left in the drawer, and indicate the number to be added. This number will be used for billing purposes.

▶ Each medication must be packaged separately and labeled with the medication name, dose, expiration date, lot number, and directions (may use sig codes, such as 1 bid, since the doses are to be given by the nursing staff).

▶ Package medications in small vials or small plastic bags, label appropriately, and place in the correct patient's medication drawer. The medication does not need to be labeled with the patient name.

▶ When the drawer contains all the required medications for the correct patient, replace it in the cassette.

▶ When the cassettes have been filled, they will be checked by a pharmacist.

▶ They can then be taken to the nursing home and exchanged with the cassettes in the medication carts.

▶ The cart exchange is often the responsibility of a technician.

Medication List for Nursing Home Patients

Patient Name	Hosp. Number	Room Number	Orders	Daily	Amt in Drawer	Amount Added
Smith, Jenny	46232-8	101-1	Ferrous Sulfate 325 mg qd		3	
			Docusate Sod 100 mg qd		1	
			Warfarin 7.5 mg bid		0	
			Propranolol 40 mg bid		2	
Savon, David	46080-5	103-2	Cimetidine 300 mg 3 bid		8	
			Bisacodyl 5 mg qhs		0	
			Acetaminophen 650 mg q4h		10	
			Methyldopa 250 mg tid		0	

Patient Name	Hosp. Number	Room Number	Orders	Daily	Amt in Drawer	Amount Added
Germain, Matilda	45201-3	101-2	**Doxycycline 100 mg q12h**		2	
			Pseudoephedrine 60 mg bid		1	
			Docusate sodium 100 mg qd		2	
			Furosemide 40 mg qd		0	
Salmon, Jerome	45681-2	102-1	**Antacid tablets 1 tid pc**		3	
			Diphenhydramine 25 mg qid		2	
			Cephalexin 500 mg qid X 10 days		0	
			Ibuprofen 200 mg qid		6	
			Multivitamin 1 qd		1	

Automated Medication Dispensing System

Medication safety is the most important factor in the practice of pharmacy. New technologies are constantly being developed to facilitate this aspect of pharmaceutical care. Technicians play a vital role in accurate medication dispensing. Most automated medication dispensing devices are maintained and serviced by technicians. This exercise will discuss the use of one technological device marketed by the Pyxis company, MedStation SN.

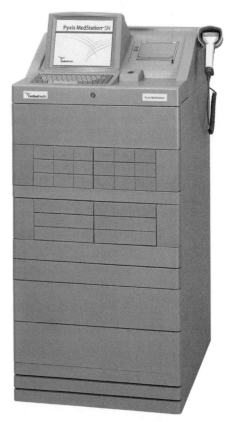

Because most training programs will not have an automated dispensing device present in the laboratory, this exercise will describe the steps involved in one of the most common functions performed by technicians in a setting using this device. It will familiarize the student with some basic procedures that can be reinforced with hands-on experience in a practice setting.

The dispensing system is a point of use system that automates the distribution, sorting, and tracking of medications. Each system, strategically located on patient floors, is connected to and communicates with a pharmacy console located in the main pharmacy.

Each system has a touch screen, a keyboard, and a printer. The types of drawers included in the system may vary according to the medications being stored. The system shown in the figure contains several types of drawers. Matrix drawers allow access to many drugs at one time because they contain open pockets suitable for "fast movers" not requiring a high degree of security. "CUBIE" drawers consist of tamper-evident portable pockets, each having a secure lid. These pockets are called "smart pockets" because they are secure medication trays embedded with an electronic chip containing information about the contents of the drawer. These drawers would be appropriate for medications requiring high control such as oral morphine or fentanyl patches.

The following is a step-by step procedure for performing the refill function in a Pyxis Medstation:

Steps:

▶ A refill report can be printed from the pharmacy console that will list the medications needing to be refilled. (A report is usually printed when the quantity in the pocket reaches a predetermined level, such as 25%.)

▶ Assume 10 fentanyl patches need to be refilled at one of the Pyxis stations.

▶ After printing the refill report, follow the Policy and Procedure Manual for the practice setting to obtain the 10 fentanyl patches.

▶ At the Medstation, touch the screen to begin.

▶ Enter User ID and Password.

▶ You will see the sections of the screen that you have access to.

▶ Touch the "Refill" button on the screen.

▶ Select the medication you want to fill by typing in the first 3 to 4 letters and then touching the appropriate medication on the screen.

▶ Touch the "Refill Selections" button on the screen to refill the selected medication.

▶ The correct drawer will open. Count the fentanyl patches in the pocket, and enter the number in the beginning count window.

▶ Press the "Accept" button on the screen.

▶ Place the 10 patches in the pocket.

▶ Enter a 10 in the refill quantity screen, and press "Accept."

▶ Enter the earliest expiration date of the patches in the drawer, and touch "Accept."

▶ Close the drawer, and the refill is complete.

The Pyxis Medstation has a tutorial that can be accessed on the touch screen for further practice, if authorized by your clinical site.

▶ Post-Lab Analysis

1. What types of drugs are usually stored in a "CUBIE" drawer in the Pyxis Medstation?

2. Discuss the importance of logging out of any pharmacy computer system after completing your task.

_____

_____

3. A discrepancy has been reported in one of the automated dispensing machines that you filled earlier in the day. List the procedures you would have followed when refilling the machine that would assure that you will not be considered at fault for the discrepancy.

_____

_____

_____

4. When filling the medication carts for a local nursing home, you notice that one of the residents has not used any of the medications sent last week. Which of the following would you do (circle one)?
   a. Add another 7 days of medication to the drawer and return it to the cart.
   b. Add no medicine to the drawer and return it to the cart.
   c. Check with the nurse on the patient's unit to see if the patient is still a resident.
   d. Remove the patient's name from the drawer and assume the patient is no longer a resident.

5. Describe computer order entry and discuss the advantages it would offer in elimination of medication errors.

_____

_____

_____

6. List three ways that technological advances can improve medication safety.

_____

_____

_____

7. List three things a technician can do to improve medication safety.

_____

_____

_____

UNIT **II**

Extemporaneous Compounds

CHAPTER 6

Prescription Balances: Torsion and Electronic

OBJECTIVES

▶ Label the parts of a torsion and an electronic balance.

▶ Explain the function of each part.

▶ Perform the leveling procedure for both types of balances.

▶ Demonstrate the calibration of a torsion balance.

▶ Tare an electronic balance.

▶ Accurately weigh a substance on each of the two types of balances.

▶ Select appropriate weighing equipment and devices for the intended purpose.

▶ Demonstrate proper cleaning and maintenance of equipment to preserve accuracy.

Extemporaneous compounding has become increasingly important as more patients and physicians are becoming aware of the possibility of compounding patient-specific products to more accurately meet the therapeutic needs of the patient. Most of this compounding will become a technician responsibility, and this offers an exciting dimension to the technician practice. Competent, accurate use of prescription balances is a vitally important aspect of prescription compounding and should be assessed on a regular basis. The following questions will help develop a basic understanding of the process before beginning hands-on practice.

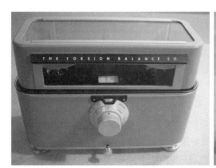 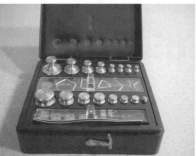 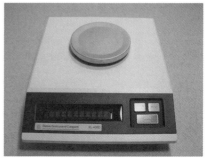

▶ Pre-Lab Questions

Using the following diagram of a torsion prescription balance as a reference, answer the questions below to demonstrate an understanding of the textbook description of the balance.

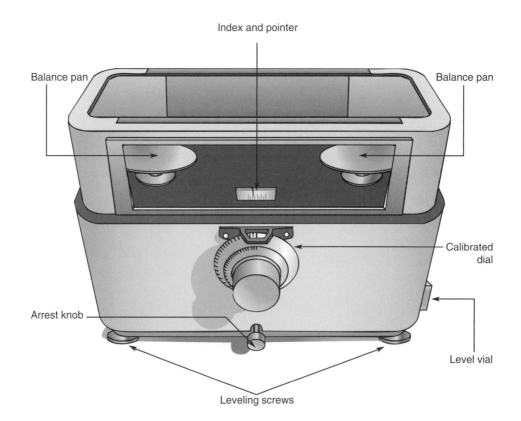

Index and pointer

Balance pan

Balance pan

Calibrated dial

Arrest knob

Level vial

Leveling screws

1. Describe the calibrated weight dial and the two calibrated scales on the dial. One scale is calibrated in the metric system. What system is the calibration of the other scale?

   _____

   _____

   _____

2. When is it appropriate to use the calibrated weight dial instead of or in addition to the prescription weights?

   _____

   _____

   _____

3. When adding the substance to be weighed to the weighing boat that has been placed on the weighing pan, should the arrest knob be open or locked? Why?

   _____

   _____

   _____

4. When using the calibrated dial, will the calibrated weight be added to the right or left side of the balance? Should the substance to be weighed be added to the right or left pan of the balance?

   _____

   _____

5. What is the sensitivity requirement of a Class III prescription balance? Describe what this means in terms of weighing accuracy.

   _____

   _____

   _____

6. The capacity of a Class III prescription balance is 15.5 grams. What does this mean in terms of the amount of powder that can be weighed on the balance?

   _____

   _____

7. An electronic single-pan balance has a sensitivity of 1 mg; some may have a capacity of 100 to 210 grams. Describe what this means in terms of the amount of powder that can accurately be weighed on an electronic balance.

_____

_____

8. Why must the prescription weights be picked up with the tweezers in the weight box and not the hands?

_____

_____

9. Why should the lid on both the torsion balance and the electronic balance be closed when leveling or taring (zeroing) the balance?

_____

_____

10. When using the leveling screws on each side to level the balance, should the screws be turned clockwise or counter-clockwise to lower the side of the balance being manipulated?

_____

▶ Lab Exercises

Most state boards of pharmacy consider the Class III prescription balance required equipment for a pharmacy department. However, many pharmacies where compounding is an important component of the practice use an electronic balance to improve speed and accuracy. Therefore, it is imperative that the technician develop some proficiency in the use of both types of balances.

Exercise 1

Weigh 5.3 grams of the indicated powder in a weighing boat on a torsion balance.

Steps:

- ▶ Place the balance on a clean flat surface away from air vents or open windows.
- ▶ Check the balance pans for any residue.
- ▶ Set the calibration dial to zero.
- ▶ Place a weighing boat in the center of each pan.
- ▶ Open the arrest knob, and check the index and pointer to see if the balance is leveled.
- ▶ If the pointer is not in the center of the index, carefully rotate the leveling screws in the correct direction to bring the pointer to a level position. Lock the arrest knob.
- ▶ Turn the calibration dial to the 0.3-g mark on the metric scale of the dial.
- ▶ Using the tweezers in the weight box, add the 5-g weight to the boat on the **right side** of the balance.
- ▶ With the arrest knob still in the locked position, add a small amount of powder to the weighing boat on the **left side** of the balance
- ▶ Unlock the arrest knob, and observe the balance pointer to determine if the amount of powder added was too little or too much.
- ▶ If the pointer rests to the left of the index center, too much powder has been added, and some needs to be removed. If the pointer is to the right of the center, too little powder has been added.
- ▶ Lock the arrest knob, and add or remove powder opening and closing the arrest knob with each addition or deletion to check the balance. When the pointer is near equilibrium, it will move back and forth within the index when the arrest knob is released. At this point, you may leave the knob unlocked and add minute amounts of powder by placing a small amount of powder on the spatula and gently tapping the spatula until the balance reaches equilibrium as indicated by the pointer remaining in the center of the index.
- ▶ Arrest the knob, and remove the weighing boat with the powder. Label the boat with the weighed powder by placing it in the assigned area on a piece of paper with your initials, the name of the powder, and 5.3 g weighed on torsion balance.
- ▶ Replace the weight and tweezers in the weight box, and close the lid. Clean the balance and pans of any residue, and close the lid. Clean residue from the spatula and proceed to the next part of the exercise.

Exercise 2

Weigh 5.3 grams of the indicated powder in a weighing boat on a digital electronic balance.

Steps:

▶ Place the balance on a clean flat surface away from air vents or open windows.

▶ Check the balance pan for any residue.

▶ Plug the balance into an outlet, and turn it on.

▶ Press the tare button. The digital display should read 0.000 g.

▶ If the numbers on the digital display are changing, the balance is being affected by movement or air currents. Close the lid.

▶ Place a weighing boat in the center of the weighing pan.

▶ Press the tare button again to zero out the weight of the boat. The digital display should again read 0.000 g.

▶ Using a spatula, add the powder to the balance pan until 5.300 g appears on the digital display. The approximate quantity to add may be determined by a visual examination of the 5.3 g previously weighed using the torsion balance and then adding small increments until the display reads 5.300 g.

▶ Remove the boat containing the weighed powder, and label it with your name, the name of the powder, and 5.3 g weighed on electronic balance.

Exercise 3

Steps:

▶ Using the same steps listed earlier for each balance, weigh the boat containing the powder originally weighed on the torsion balance by placing it on the electronic balance pan. Tare the balance first using an empty weighing boat.

▶ Record the weight: _____. Record the weight also under your original notation as weight recorded from electronic balance.

▶ Using the steps outlined for the torsion balance, place the boat containing the powder weighed on the electronic balance on the left side pan of the torsion balance.

▶ Place an empty weighing boat on the right side pan, and add weight to the right side of the balance using weights and the calibrated dial. Record the weight: _____. Record the weight also on the paper with your name and original notations as weight determined by torsion balance.

▶ Place both pans in the area designated by your instructor for checking.

▶ Post-Lab Analysis

1. Jim works in a pharmacy where extemporaneous compounding is not often required. It has been several months since he last used the Class III torsion prescription balance available in the pharmacy. He placed the balance on a flat surface and leveled it. He needed 5.3 g of dextrose powder, so he placed a weighing boat on each balance pan and added a 5-g weight to the left side pan. He decided to use the calibration dial for the additional 0.3 g needed, so he carefully set the metric scale to 0.3 g. He then began to carefully add powder to the boat on the right side of the balance, arresting and releasing the knob between each addition until the pointer rested in the center of the index. What concern do you have about the accuracy of the powder weight? Why? What would you expect to be the actual weight of the powder weighed by Jim?

   _____

   _____

   _____

   _____

2. A torsion balance has a sensitivity of 6 mg. The generally accepted margin of error for weighing compounding ingredients is 5%. To avoid a margin of error above 5%, what is the minimum quantity that should be weighed on a torsion balance? Show your work in the blank space below and circle the answer.

3. Describe any variance in the weight of your powders on the two different scales. What could account for variations.

   _____

   _____

4. Discuss the advantages and disadvantages of the two types of scales used.

   _____

   _____

CHAPTER 7

Dry Powders for External Use

OBJECTIVES

▶ Demonstrate the methods for reducing particle size of powders for topical preparations.

▶ Blend two or more powders together to form a homogenous mixture.

▶ Reduce particle size using a mesh sieve.

▶ Use geometric dilution to combine unequal amounts of powders.

▶ Properly package and label a dusting powder preparation for dispensing.

TERMS

Comminution

Trituration

Blending

Tumbling

100-mesh sieve

Geometric dilution

Particle size

Homogenous mixture

Eutectic mixture

Dusting powder

EQUIPMENT AND INGREDIENTS

Class III prescription torsion

Balance or electronic balance

Mortars/pestles

Glassine papers or weighing

Boats

Spatulas

Ointment papers or slab

Menthol

Starch

Salicylic acid

Shaker top dispenser

Ziploc® plastic bags

Mesh sieve

For compounding purposes, powders need to be in a state of fine, evenly sized particles. If they cannot be purchased in this form, there are several methods of processing them to produce the necessary particle size. When more than one powder is to be combined, the chemicals must be blended to a homogenous mixture. Reduction of particle size is often accomplished with the use of a mortar and pestle. The photograph depicts the three types of mortars and pestles commonly used in pharmaceutical compounding (glass, wedgewood, and ceramic).

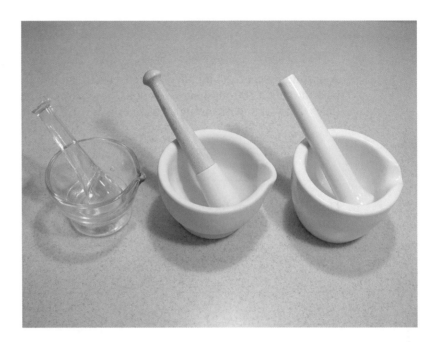

▶ Pre-Lab Questions

1. List three important factors to be considered when compounding a bulk powder for external application.

   _____

   _____

   _____

   _____

2. Discuss the importance of uniform particle size when compounding bulk powders.

   _____

   _____

3. When a dusting powder contains an active ingredient, what effect does particle size have on the topical effect of the active ingredient?

_____

_____

4. The process of reducing particle size of solids is called comminution. Name two techniques used to accomplish comminution of a solid substance.

_____

_____

5. A dusting powder should have particles small enough that 50% of the particles will pass through a 100-mesh sieve. Would these particles be larger or smaller than particles that would pass through a 50-mesh sieve? Explain.

_____

_____

6. Discuss the reasons for choosing each of the different types of mortars and pestles in terms of the type of surface and their effectiveness in trituration of various chemicals.

_____

_____

_____

_____

_____

7. After an acceptable particle size has been achieved, it is important to create a homogenous mixture. Name four methods for accomplishing this.

_____

_____

_____

_____

8. Describe the process of geometric dilution.

_____

_____

_____

_____

▶ Lab Exercises

*Compound the following prescription using the following two different methods. Record ingredients and compounding techniques on a **Master Formula Sheet.***

James Anderson, MD
2901 Church Street, Brooks, IN 47604
Phone: (356) 443-0098 Fax: (356) 444-9800

Name: Sammy Smitz   **Date:** 05-03-07

Address: 2603 South Hampshire Road, Brooks, IN 53706

RX: Menthol   .1 grams
Salicylic Acid .1 grams
Starch   qs AD 30 grams
SIG. Apply To callous on Bottom f Feet Daily

Refills 3

James Anderson, MD

_____   _____
Dispense as written   May substitute

Method 1

Force the eutectic mixture to liquefy, and adsorb it with the starch.

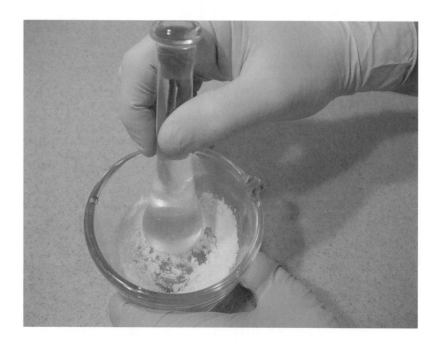

Steps:

1. Weigh each of the ingredients using either a prescription torsion balance or an electronic scale.

2. Combine the menthol and the salicylic acid in a glass mortar and mix with the pestle until they liquefy.

3. Triturate the starch with a wedgewood mortar and pestle to reduce any particles that may have clumped together during transportation and storage of the manufactured product.

4. Using geometric dilution, place an amount of starch powder approximately equal to the liquefied amount of the eutectic mixture into the glass mortar and triturate, allowing the eutectic mixture to adsorb on the starch.

5. Continue adding an amount of the starch equal to the amount of the mixture in the glass mortar, triturating after each addition to form a homogenous mixture, until all the starch has been added. Triturate until the mixture is blended into a fine homogenous powder.

6. Place the powder in a mesh sieve to determine the fineness of the particles. If necessary, triturate the powders again to achieve a fine homogenous powder suitable for topical application. Weigh the final product to assure accuracy.

7. Place the powder in a plastic container with a shaker top for ease of application for the patient.

8. Enter the required data in the **Master Formula Sheet**.

9. Type a label for the prescription, including either amounts or percentages of each ingredient.

10. Apply the correct auxiliary label and a 3-month expiration date.

11. Organize the ingredients used, the final product, and the **Master Formula Sheet** for the instructor to check.

Method 2

Using a protectant to prevent liquefaction of eutectic chemicals:

Steps:

1. Weigh each of the ingredients separately on either a prescription torsion balance or an electronic balance.

2. Triturate each of the chemicals separately with a mortar and pestle until each is a fine powder.

3. Use an amount of starch equal to the amount of salicylic acid as a protectant. Triturate the starch and salicylic acid until blended and a fine homogenous mixture is formed.

4. Triturate an amount of starch equal to the amount of menthol until the mixture is blended into a fine homogenous mixture.

5. Combine the starch-salicylic acid mixture, the starch-menthol mixture, and an amount of starch equal to the combination of those two mixtures and continue to triturate, using a spatula to remove powder from the sides of the mortar and assure a homogenous mixture.

6. Using geometric dilution, continue adding starch to the mixture and triturating after each addition.

7. When all the starch has been added, continue to triturate and use a spatula to move powder from the sides of the mortar back to the center until the entire mixture is a homogenous blend of fine particles.

8. Pass the mixture through a mesh sieve to assure a fine particle size.

9. Weigh the final product to assure the total weight is accurate.

10. Place the final product in a plastic shaker top container for ease of application by the patient.

11. Record the necessary data in the **Master Formula Sheet**.

12. Enter the compound in the computer, and apply a prescription label to the container.

13. Add the appropriate auxiliary label and a 3-month expiration date.

14. Leave the product, ingredients used, and **Master Formula Sheet** with the prescription for checking by the instructor.

▶ Post-Lab Analysis

1. Describe the interaction that might have occurred if the menthol, salicylic acid, and starch had been mixed together in one step.

   _____

   _____

   _____

2. Define the term "protectant" as demonstrated in Method 2. Discuss the properties of the starch that caused it to be a suitable protectant.

   _____

   _____

3. What action would you expect salicylic acid to have in this preparation?

   _____

4. What adverse effect might occur if the salicylic acid was not homogenously distributed in the topical powder?

   _____

   _____

5. What topical effects would be expected from the menthol in this preparation?

   _____

6. Which of the two compounding methods did you prefer and why?

   _____

   _____

7. Was there a difference in the appearance or texture of the two final products? If so, explain.

   _____

   _____

MASTER FORMULA SHEET

Compound _____ Quantity _____ Exp Date _____

Student Name _____ Instructor _____ Date _____

INGREDIENT	NDC #	LOT #	QUANTITY	EXP DATE
Notes:				

MASTER FORMULA SHEET

Compound _____ Quantity _____ Exp Date _____

Student Name _____ Instructor _____ Date _____

INGREDIENT	NDC #	LOT #	QUANTITY	EXP DATE
Notes:				

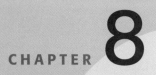

CHAPTER **8**

Capsules

OBJECTIVES

▶ Discuss the advantages of extemporaneously compounded capsules.

▶ Demonstrate the ability to prepare an aliquot when the amount of drug needed is below the 120-mg minimum accuracy for the balance.

▶ Determine the amount of filler needed and the correct capsule size for a formulation.

▶ Compound capsules using the punch method and a simple capsule-filling device.

▶ Pre-Lab Questions

1. Describe a hard-shell gelatin capsule, including the terms body, cap, and capsule size.

   _____

   _____

   _____

2. Discuss the punch method of preparing capsules.

   _____

   _____

   _____

3. List several ways to accomplish uniform dispersion of powders before filling capsules.

   _____

   _____

   _____

4. How can food coloring be used to aid in assuring complete dispersion of powders?

   _____

   _____

5. List two advantages of extemporaneously compounded capsules as a dosage form.

   _____

   _____

   _____

6. Name two disadvantages of capsules as a dosage form.

   _____

   _____

7. A prescription ordered 5 mg of quinine sulfate powder per dose to be added to diphen-hydramine powder and dispensed in a capsule. The quantity to dispense is 12 capsules. The total quantity of quinine sulfate needed for the order is 60 mg. This is below the minimum amount that can be accurately weighed on a prescription balance. Describe the process for making an acceptable aliquot, and show the calculations.

_____

_____

_____

_____

▶ Lab Exercises

Using the following prescription, follow the steps outlined below and fill in the appropriate data as required.

Michael Angelo, D.O.
806 Cherry Creek Plaza, Denver, CO 50620
702-317-5030

Name: Sally Sue Sullivan   **Date:** _____ 10/19/06 _____

Address: 6072 Denver West Dr., Boulder, CO

RX: Acetominophen   325mg
       Ibuprofen   100 mg
       mix and prepare 12 capsules

Sig: Give one capsule qid for pain and fever

_____   *Michael Angelo, D.O.* _____

Dispense as written   May substitute

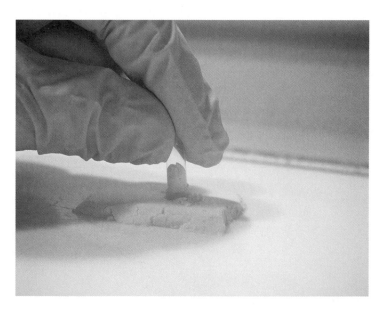

Hand-filling a capsule with dry powder using the punch method.

Hand Filling a Capsule

Steps:

Prepare materials for 2 extra capsules to account for powder loss.

1. Available materials: acetaminophen 325 mg tablets, ibuprofen powder, and dextrose powder.

2. Number of acetaminophen tablets needed for the preparation _____.

3. Weigh acetaminophen tablets to determine amount of drug plus filler.

4. Amount of ibuprofen needed for preparation _____.

5. Place acetaminophen tablets into a mortar and triturate with pestle until reduced to a fine powder.

6. Weigh ibuprofen powder.

7. Add a few drops of food color to ibuprofen powder, and mix until color is even.

8. Determine amount of dextrose powder needed to fill 12 number 0 capsules plus 2 extra to account for powder loss during compounding _____.

9. Weigh dextrose powder.

10. Begin mixing colored ibuprofen powder with acetaminophen and dextrose powder using geometric dilution and trituration.

11. Scrape sides of mortar frequently, and continue mixing until color is even.

12. Pass the powder mixture through a fine mesh sieve to obtain a uniform distribution of particle sizes.

13. Place the powder on a powder paper and, using a spatula, form a smooth block that is about $\frac{1}{2}$ the length of the capsule body.

14. Wearing gloves to prevent hand contact, separate 14 capsules and place them in an empty weighing boat.

15. Begin "punching" the capsules by taking the body of a capsule and holding it in an upright position. Punch the open end repeatedly into the powder until full.

16. Replace the capsule cap and weigh each capsule using an empty capsule on the other pan of the balance or tare an electronic balance with an empty capsule on the pan. Weight must be between 90% and 110% of calculated weight.

17. Clean capsules with a soft tissue and place in appropriate container. Label, including expiration date, and leave with appropriate paperwork for the final check.

Capsule Compounding Using a Capsule-Filling Device

Steps:

1. Repeat steps 1–13 under *Hand Filling a Capsule*.
2. Load capsule-filling device with the body of the capsules to be filled.
3. Place weighed powder on device over capsules. Using spatula provided, spread powder over capsules until they are filled. Tamp the powder into the capsules with a glass stirring rod or capsule tamper.
4. Place caps on capsules and weigh to check for accuracy and uniformity.
5. Repeat step 18 under *Hand Filling a Capsule*.

▶ Post-Lab Analysis

1. Discuss the two methods of capsule filling in terms of achieving accuracy and uniformity of capsule weight.

   _____

   _____

   _____

   _____

2. Discuss the two methods of capsule filling in terms of speed and difficulty.

   _____

   _____

   _____

   _____

3. Tell which of the two methods of capsule filling you would prefer for a prescription requiring 12 compounded capsules, and give reasons for your answer.

   _____

   _____

   _____

   _____

   _____

4. Tell which of the two methods of capsule filling you would prefer if compounding a prescription calling for 100 capsules, and give reasons for your answer.

_____

_____

_____

_____

5. How did you determine the expiration date for the capsules compounded in this exercise?

_____

_____

MASTER FORMULA SHEET

Compound _____ Quantity _____ Exp Date _____

Student Name _____ Instructor _____ Date _____

INGREDIENT	NDC #	LOT #	QUANTITY	EXP DATE
Notes:				

MASTER FORMULA SHEET

Compound _____ Quantity _____ Exp Date _____

Student Name _____ Instructor _____ Date _____

INGREDIENT	NDC #	LOT #	QUANTITY	EXP DATE
Notes:				

CHAPTER 9

Solutions and Syrups

OBJECTIVES

▶ Discuss the advantages of oral solutions as a dosage form.

▶ List the physical characteristics of common solvents.

▶ Discuss methods of facilitating solution.

▶ Demonstrate the ability to compound various types of solutions.

▶ Evaluate the compounded solutions and syrups for pharmaceutical elegance.

TERMS

Spirits
Tinctures
Elixirs
Syrups
Otic solutions
Nasal solutions
Ophthalmic solutions
Vehicle
Solvent
Solute
Saturated solution
Eutectic mixture
Solubility
Flavoring agent

EQUIPMENT AND INGREDIENTS

Graduates
Mortars/pestles
Stirring rods
Prescription balance/electronic balance
Prescription weights
Glycerin
Hydrogen peroxide
Coal tar
Tincture of green soap
Loratidine syrup
Acetaminophen drops or liquid
Sodium chloride
Boric acid (crystals or powder)
Ora-Sweet

Solutions are clear, homogenous liquids in which a drug is completely dissolved. They may be used topically, as inhalations, parenterally, or as oral dosage forms. This chapter includes extemporaneous compounds of both topical and oral solutions. Parenteral solutions will be covered in another chapter.

▶ Pre-Lab Questions

1. Name three methods for speeding up the solution of a solute in a solvent.

   _____

   _____

   _____

2. List three advantages of solutions.

   _____

   _____

   _____

3. List the disadvantages of solutions.

   _____

   _____

   _____

4. List one ingredient that will always be in a true elixir.

   _____

5. What effect (s) would hydrogen peroxide have in an ear preparation?

   _____

6. What would be the purpose of the glycerin in a mixture of hydrogen peroxide and glycerin to be placed in the ear?

   _____

   _____

7. Describe the meniscus, and describe how it is used in measuring liquids.

   _____

   _____

   _____

8. Define a saturated solution. What would you expect to happen if you added more solute to a saturated solution?

_____

_____

9. Name the three most common vehicles for pharmaceutical solutions.

_____

▶ Lab Exercises

Follow the weighing techniques outlined in Chapter 6 to weigh the dry ingredients for the compounds in the following prescriptions. Accuracy in measuring liquids is vital to preparing a solution that meets the specifications of the prescription ordered by the prescriber. Practice the liquid measuring techniques listed below before preparing the compounds. Step-by-step instructions for each compound follow the prescriptions.

In the blanks next to each prescription, note any calculations or any action needed.

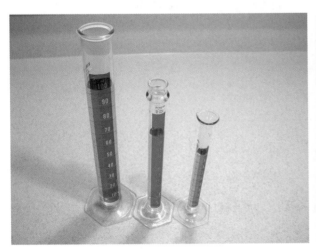
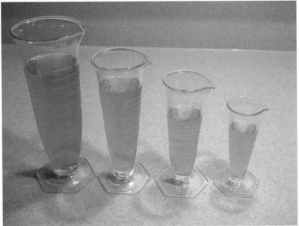

Liquid Measuring Techniques

Steps:

▶ Cylindrical graduates have sides that are parallel to each other and perpendicular to the base. They should have graduation marks that are clear and distinct in either milliliters or ounces. Quantities below 2 ml (the smallest cylindrical graduate available is 10 ml) should be measured with an oral syringe.

▶ Conical graduates are circular graduates with sides that flare out from the base. They should not be used if they have a capacity of less than 15 ml.

▶ Other measuring devices include 1- and 3-ml oral syringes and calibrated or uncalibrated eyedroppers.

▶ The general rule when measuring liquids for extemporaneous compounding is to measure a volume that is at least 20% of the total volume capacity of the measuring device to minimize the potential for error. Use the smallest measuring device that will accommodate the amount to be measured.

▶ Liquids poured into a container will form a concave-shaped surface called a meniscus. When reading the volume of the liquid, the bottom of the meniscus and the graduation mark on the container should be aligned with the direct line of sight. In other words, hold the graduate up to eye level to read the graduation mark.

Prescriptions

PRESCRIPTION 9.1

Joseph VanMeter, MD
8012 Chelsea, Indianapolis, IN 46203

Jimmy Smith   1-20-04

806 Winding Way, Indianapolis, IN 46220   **Age:** 10

RX: Glycerin   15ml
         Hydrogen Peroxide 3% solution 15ml
         Mix well and dispense in a dropper bottle

Sig: 3g tt au gid prn earache

Refill 1X

_____   Joseph VanMeter, MD
Dispense as written   May substitute

PRESCRIPTION 9.2

Charles Silva, MD, License #830361
604 West 3rd Street, Carmel, IN 46702

Sam Houston   1-20-04

611 Terrace Way, Fishers, IN 46578

RX: Coal Tar Solution 5%
Tincture Green Soap qs ad 60 ml

Sig: Apply to scalp 3X per week

Refill 3 times

_____   *Charles Silva, MD*
Dispense as written   May substitute

PRESCRIPTION 9.3

John White, MD
604 West 3rd Street, Suite 5, Carmel, IN

Sandy Jones   1-20-04

1211 North Colwater Road, Indianapolis, IN 46306

RX: Boric Acid 3% Solution
120 ml

Sig: Rinse affected area bid

_____   *John White, MD*
Dispense as written   May substitute

PRESCRIPTION 9.4

Thomas Myer, DO
1812 College Way, Okemos, MI 68430
(503)863-4707

Nathan Jones   **Date:** 6-24-05

6245 Derbyshire Drive, Holt, MI 68452

RX: Loratidine 1mg/5cc
Acetaminophen 120 mg/5cc
Ora-Sweet qs ad 60 ml

Sig: Give 5cc (one teaspoonful) bid prn cold
symptoms.

_____   *Thomas Myer, DO*
Dispense as written   May substitute

PRESCRIPTION 9.5

Thomas Myer, DO
1812 College Way, Okemos, MI 68430
(503)863-4707

Nathan Jones   **Date:** 6-24-05

6245 Derbyshire Drive, Holt, MI 68452

RX: Normal Saline Nose Drops

            30 ml

Sig: Place 2-3 drops in each nostril Bid
            Followed. By suction with a nasal
                        sponge

_____   Thomas Myer, DO
Dispense as written   May substitute

Compounding Instructions

Steps for Prescription 9.1: Glycerin-Hydrogen Peroxide Solution

1. Select the appropriate size graduate to measure each of the two liquids.
2. Combine the two liquids, and mix well with a glass stirring rod.
3. Pour mixture into a 1-ounce dropper bottle.
4. Enter data into software system, and affix label to bottle. Add needed auxiliary labels.
5. Fill out the **Master Formula Sheet** and leave ingredients used, paperwork, and final product for pharmacist to check
6. Clean all lab equipment used, and return to proper place.

Steps for Prescription 9.2:
Coal Tar-Tincture Green Soap Solution:

1. Calculate the amount of Coal Tar Solution needed.

2. Measure Coal Tar Solution using either a glass graduate or a disposable oral syringe.

3. Transfer the Coal Tar Solution to a glass cylindrical or conical graduate with a capacity of 60 ml or more.

4. Add a sufficient quantity of Tincture of Green Soap to bring the bottom of the meniscus to the 60-ml graduation mark.

4. Stir the mixture with a glass stirring rod. Do not shake.

5. Pour mixture into a 2-ounce prescription bottle.

6. Enter data into the prescription software system, and affix the label to the bottle. Add any needed auxiliary labels.

7. Fill out the **Master Formula Sheet** and leave ingredients used, paperwork, and final product for the pharmacist to check.

8. Clean all lab equipment used, and return to appropriate place in the lab.

Steps for Prescription 9.3: Boric Acid 3% Solution

1. Calculate the amount of boric acid needed for a 3% solution.

2. Check an appropriate reference book for the solubility of boric acid to be sure a 3% solution is feasible.

3. Weigh the boric acid powder (or crystals) on the electronic or the torsion balance.

4. Place boric acid in a conical graduate.

5. Measure 120 ml of water in a cylindrical graduate.

6. Add the water to the boric acid in the conical graduate until the meniscus reaches the 120-ml graduated mark.

7. Measure and make note of the amount of water left in the cylindrical graduate.

8. Mix the boric acid with a glass stirring rod until completely dissolved and no crystals are seen floating in the solution. (May use a heated water bath if available.)

9. Pour mixture into a 4-ounce bottle.

10. Enter data into the prescription software system, and affix the label to the bottle. Add any needed auxiliary labels.

11. Fill out the **Master Formula Sheet** and leave ingredients used, paperwork, and final product for the pharmacist to check.

12. Clean all lab equipment used, and return to appropriate place in the lab.

Steps for Prescription 9.4:
Loratidine-Acetaminophen Solution

1. Calculate the amounts of loratidine syrup and acetaminophen liquid needed to provide the correct concentration.
2. Measure each using a measuring device appropriate for the amounts to be measured.
3. Mix the two syrups together in a graduate with at least a 60-ml capacity.
4. Add a sufficient quantity of Ora-Sweet to reach the 60-ml graduation mark.
5. Mix well with a glass stirring rod, and pour into a 2-ounce bottle.
6. Enter data into the prescription software system, and affix the label to the bottle. Add any needed auxiliary labels. Dispense with appropriate measuring device for administration.
7. Fill out the **Master Formula Sheet** and leave ingredients used, paperwork, and final product for the pharmacist to check.
8. Clean all lab equipment used, and return to appropriate place in the lab.

Steps for Prescription 9.5: Normal Saline Nose Drops

1. Calculate the amount of sodium chloride needed to compound 30 ml of normal saline.
2. Weigh the appropriate amount of sodium chloride.
3. Dissolve sodium chloride in 30 ml of water.
4. Pour solution into a 1-ounce dropper bottle.
5. Enter data into the prescription software system, and affix the label to the bottle. Add any needed auxiliary labels.
6. Fill out the **Master Formula Sheet** and leave ingredients used, paperwork, and final product for the pharmacist to check.
7. Clean all lab equipment used, and return to appropriate place in the lab.

▶ Post-Lab Analysis

1. Which of the prescriptions prepared in the Steps require the "For External Use Only" label?

   _____

   _____

2. What measuring device should be used to measure the Coal Tar Solution? Why is this the best choice?

   _____

   _____

3. Give a possible use for the Coal Tar-Tincture of Green Soap solution.

_____

_____

4. What would be the purpose of placing saline drops in the nostril and then suctioning with a nasal syringe?

_____

_____

5. Which two liquid formulations of acetaminophen liquid would be appropriate for obtaining the required strength indicated in the loratidine-acetaminophen prescription?

_____

_____

6. Calculate the amounts that would be needed for each of the two acetaminophen formulations in question 5. Show calculations in the space below. Be sure to label your answers.

_____

7. What age child would this preparation be appropriate for in terms of dose?

_____

8. What would be the advantage of combining the two ingredients?

_____

_____

9. How often is loratidine usually dosed in a 24-hour period?

_____

_____

10. Boric acid solution is a weak anti-infective sometimes used to cleanse delicate tissue. List two serious toxic effects that might occur if ingested by a child.

_____

_____

11. What auxiliary label(s) would be required on this preparation?

_____

_____

12. If the Boric acid prescription had called for 30 ml of a 0.1% solution of boric acid, how would you prepare this solution? The amount of boric acid needed would be less than the least amount that can be accurately weighed on a prescription balance. Discuss the procedure for making a liquid aliquot. Show calculations and label answers.

_____

_____

MASTER FORMULA SHEET

Compound _____ Quantity _____ Exp Date _____

Student Name _____ Instructor _____ Date _____

INGREDIENT	NDC #	LOT #	QUANTITY	EXP DATE
Notes:				

MASTER FORMULA SHEET

Compound _____ Quantity _____ Exp Date _____

Student Name _____ Instructor _____ Date _____

INGREDIENT	NDC #	LOT #	QUANTITY	EXP DATE
Notes:				

MASTER FORMULA SHEET

Compound _____ Quantity _____ Exp Date _____

Student Name _____ Instructor _____ Date _____

INGREDIENT	NDC #	LOT #	QUANTITY	EXP DATE

Notes:

MASTER FORMULA SHEET

Compound _____ Quantity _____ Exp Date _____

Student Name _____ Instructor _____ Date _____

INGREDIENT	NDC #	LOT #	QUANTITY	EXP DATE

Notes:

MASTER FORMULA SHEET

Compound _____ Quantity _____ Exp Date _____

Student Name _____ Instructor _____ Date _____

INGREDIENT	NDC #	LOT #	QUANTITY	EXP DATE
Notes:				

MASTER FORMULA SHEET

Compound _____ Quantity _____ Exp Date _____

Student Name _____ Instructor _____ Date _____

INGREDIENT	NDC #	LOT #	QUANTITY	EXP DATE
Notes:				

Suspensions and Lotions

TERMS

Powder displacement

Reconstitution

Flocculated suspending agent

Suspension

Viscosity

Therapeutic dose range

Emollient

Antipruritic

Anti-inflammatory

Pharmaceutical elegance

EQUIPMENT AND INGREDIENTS

Empty antibiotic suspension bottles

Dextrose

Food coloring

Ora Plus

Propranolol 40-mg tablets

Simple syrup

Menthol

Alcohol

Hydrocortisone cream 0.5% 30-g tubes

Lubriderm lotion

Prescription balance

Mortar and pestle

OBJECTIVES

▶ Demonstrate proper technique for reconstituting dry powders for oral suspensions.

▶ Calculate powder displacement for accurate reconstitution.

▶ Prepare an oral suspension using a flocculated suspending agent.

▶ Compound a lotion for topical use.

Many antibiotics are relatively unstable when placed in a liquid formulation. To lengthen the shelf life and still provide a liquid formulation, the antibiotic powder is packaged in a granular form requiring reconstitution. The amount of liquid required to produce 150 ml of the antibiotic suspension must include a calculation of the amount of powder displacement. Water used for reconstitution should always be distilled or purified water because tap water contains chemicals that may contaminate the preparation.

Often a product that is available commercially in a tablet dosage form is prescribed for a patient unable to swallow a tablet. Pulverization of the tablet and combining with a suspending agent yields a pharmaceutically elegant product.

Medications indicated for topical application may be formulated as a lotion.

▶ Pre-Lab Questions

1. A commercial preparation of amoxicillin powder for suspension specifies a concentration of 250 mg per 5 cc. The final volume of the preparation is to be 150 ml. If the amount of distilled water added to the container is 97 ml, what is the powder displacement in this product? Show your calculations below and circle your answer.

2. What concentration would result if the amoxicillin product above was reconstituted with 150 ml of distilled water, and what would be the final volume of the product?

3. If a dry powder for reconstitution has a final volume of 200 ml and the powder displacement is 12 ml, how much distilled water should be added to the powder to produce the appropriate concentration?

4. What auxiliary label should be applied to all suspension formulations?

   _____

5. What auxiliary label information should be included on a prescription for penicillin for oral suspension when it is dispensed?

   _____

   _____

   _____

   _____

6. How would you determine the expiration date and storage requirements for an oral suspension compounded by pulverizing tablets and adding a suspending agent to produce a liquid suspension?

_____

_____

7. What type of containers would be appropriate for dispensing a lotion compounded in the pharmacy?

_____

_____

8. What auxiliary labels should be applied to a topical lotion?

_____

_____

▶ Lab Exercises

Exercise 1

Follow the instructions below for Prescription 10.1.

PRESCRIPTION 10.1

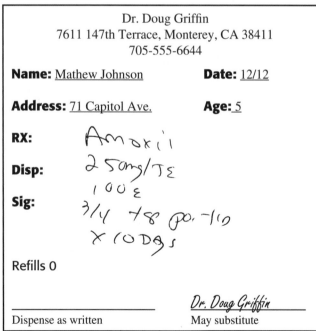

Dr. Doug Griffin
7611 147th Terrace, Monterey, CA 38411
705-555-6644

Name: Mathew Johnson   **Date:** 12/12

Address: 71 Capitol Ave.   **Age:** 5

RX: Amoxil

Disp: 250mg/T₅
            100 ₅

Sig: 3/4 +8 po. -/10
            X 10DgS

Refills 0

_____   *Dr. Doug Griffin*
Dispense as written   May substitute

Fill Prescription 10.1 by reconstitution of the amoxicillin powder for oral suspension.

Steps:

▶ Determine the correct amount of distilled water to use by checking the manufacturer's instructions on the label.

▶ Measure the correct amount of water in an appropriately sized graduate.

▶ Turn capped bottle of powder upside down and tap on counter to loosen powder from corners of bottle.

▶ Use the correct method for adding the water in two portions.

▶ Shake vigorously after each addition.

▶ Check for complete mixture of the powder with no "powder pockets" at the bottom of the bottle.

▶ If powder pockets exist, use a glass stirring rod to mix the undissolved powder.

▶ Prepare a prescription label, add appropriate auxiliary labels, and leave preparation and paperwork in the designated area for a final check.

Exercise 2

Prepare Prescription 10.2 using 40-mg tablets of propranolol. Calculate the number of 40-mg tablets needed for the preparation. Show calculations. Label and circle your answer.

PRESCRIPTION 10.2

David J. Davis, MD
2608 Manchester Court, Boston, MA, 67034

Name: Joseph James   **Date:** 6/3/05

2901 Green Apple Road, Boston, MA, 60750

RX: PROPANOLOL SUSPENSION 10mg/5cc
        120 ml

Sig: Take 5cc PO qid

Refills 1 2 3 6

_____   *David J. Davis, MD*
Dispense as written   May substitute

Steps:

‣ Triturate the tablets with a mortar and pestle until a fine powder is achieved.

‣ Add 30 ml of OraPlus, a flocculating suspending agent, and mix well. Pour into 100-ml graduate, and measure volume to determine powder displacement. QS to 100 ml with simple syrup.

‣ Pour into 4-ounce prescription bottle. Shake well, and add the 20 ml of simple syrup to bring the total quantity to 120 ml.

‣ Prepare a **Master Formula Sheet** (provided at end of chapter), indicating amount of powder displacement and liquids added, and include expiration date and storage requirements.

‣ Prepare a prescription label, and add auxiliary labels.

‣ Leave final product, in a pharmaceutically elegant condition, with appropriate auxiliary labels in the designated area for a final check.

‣ Clean lab supplies and work area.

Exercise 3

Calculate the amount of menthol needed for a 1% preparation as shown in Prescription 10.3. Show calculations in the space below. Circle and label your answer.

PRESCRIPTION 10.3

Thomas James, DO
2403 Lansing Lane, Flint, MI 68432

Name: Sally Rodgers   **Date:** 7/05/05

Address: 7403 South Pleasantview Road, Detroit, MI, 76804

RX: MENTHOL 1%
HYDROCORTISONE CREAM 0.5%
30 gm

Quantity: qs to 60 ml with LUBRIDERM

Sig: Apply to affected area bid

Thomas James, DO

Dispense as written   May substitute

Steps:

▶ Weigh menthol and transfer to mortar. Add a small amount of alcohol, and triturate until dissolved.

▶ Add a small amount of hydrocortisone cream, and triturate until well mixed. Continue adding small amount until evenly distributed.

▶ Place in conical graduate and QS with Lubriderm lotion in several additions, mixing after each addition until even mixture is obtained and 60-ml volume is reached.

▶ Transfer to appropriate container, taking care to preserve pharmaceutical elegance.

▶ Prepare a **Master Formula Sheet.**

▶ Label with prescription label and any auxiliary labels needed.

▶ Leave with paperwork in designated area for final check.

▶ Post-Lab Analysis

1. The prescription for Matthew Johnson for Amoxicillin 250/5 calls for a dose of ¾ teaspoonful three times a day for 10 days. The dose range for amoxicillin is 20 to 50 mg/kg/day in divided doses q8h. If Matthew weighs 100 pounds, would this be considered an appropriate dose? Using the following information from the package insert, calculate the dose range for a child weighing 100 pounds. Label and circle your answer.

    Pkg insert dose range: 20 mg/kg/d minimum to 40 mg/kg/d maximum
    a. Matthew's weight in kg _____
    b. Calculated dose for Matthew's weight at 20 mg/kg/d _____
       (minimum recommended dose)
    c. Calculated dose for Matthew's weight at 40 mg/kg/d _____
       (maximum recommended dose)
    d. Daily dose range for amoxicillin for Matthew's weight in mg/d _____
    e. Single dose range for Matthew's weight in mg/dose (daily dose divided by 3 doses/day) _____

2. Explain whether the dosage for Matthew Johnson given in question 1 is above, below, or in the dosage range recommended by the manufacturer.

    _____

    What would be the possible consequences of a subtherapeutic dose?

    _____

    _____

    What would be the possible consequences of a dose higher than the recommended dose?

    _____

    _____

3. In compounding the propranolol suspension in Joseph James' prescription, how many tablets would be needed for the compound if only 10-mg propranolol tablets were available? Show calculations below. Label and circle your answer.

   How could the amount of powder displacement and the amount of liquid needed be affected by using 10-mg tablets instead of 40-mg tablets? Why?

   _____

   _____

   _____

4. Describe the therapeutic effect of each of the ingredients in the topical lotion preparation.

   Menthol _____

   Hydrocortisone cream _____

   Lubriderm Lotion _____

5. What side effect might the patient experience if, in your calculations for menthol, the decimal point was moved two places to the right in error?

   _____

MASTER FORMULA SHEET

Compound _____ Quantity _____ Exp Date _____

Student Name _____ Instructor _____ Date _____

INGREDIENT	NDC #	LOT #	QUANTITY	EXP DATE
Notes:				

MASTER FORMULA SHEET

Compound _____ Quantity _____ Exp Date _____

Student Name _____ Instructor _____ Date _____

INGREDIENT	NDC #	LOT #	QUANTITY	EXP DATE
Notes:				

Ointments and Creams

OBJECTIVES

▶ Learn the rationale for topical formulations with ointment and cream bases.

▶ Know the physical characteristics of common bases used.

▶ Demonstrate compounding techniques.

▶ Experience the compounding of topical formulations.

▶ Evaluate the ointment and cream formulations for consistency and pharmaceutical elegance.

▶ **Pre-Lab Questions**

1. List three advantages of topical drug delivery.

   _____

   _____

   _____

2. List three disadvantages of topical drug delivery.

   _____

   _____

   _____

3. What is the purpose of a levigating agent?

   _____

4. Name two conditions in which an ointment preparation would be used rather than a cream, and tell why an ointment is preferable.

   _____

   _____

Fill in the blanks in questions 5, 6, 7, and 8 with the correct term from the following list.
White petrolatum   Dermabase   Mineral oil   Polyethylene glycol

5. _____ would provide an acceptable base for a preparation with good protective and occlusive properties that would not be water washable and would not absorb water.

6. _____ would provide a base that is water soluble, water washable, can absorb some water, and is nonocclusive and nongreasy.

7. An oil in water emulsion that is water washable but not water soluble is called a cream. An example of this would be _____.

8. An example of a levigating agent would be _____.

9. Dry powders may need to be triturated before adding to the ointment base because:

   _____

10. Small amounts of powders with fine, uniform particle size may be incorporated into the ointment base using the _____ technique.

▶ Lab Exercises

*Prepare the products in the following prescriptions using the proper technique as demonstrated by your instructor. Package and label each of the products, being certain to include any necessary auxiliary labels. Check your final product for pharmaceutical elegance. Document your procedure and ingredients on the **Master Formula Sheet.***

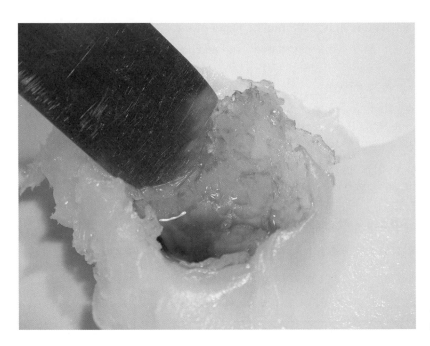

Using a depression in white petrolatum to incorporate povidone-iodine solution.

PRESCRIPTION 11.1

Joseph Sorbonne, MD
2802 E. Hardwick
Anycity, Alaska

Marie Shivvers   **Date**   10-19-06

806 North 6th Pontoon Lake, Alaska

RX: Povidone-Iodine Solution 5ml
White petrolatum   60GM
Mix & Dispense

Sig: Apply to injured area on Knee after cleaning with Peroxide bid.

_____   *Joseph Sorbonne, MD*
Dispense as written   May substitute

Steps:

1. Using the appropriate size graduate (or oral syringe), measure 5 ml of povidone-iodine solution.

2. Calibrate prescription balance and weigh 60 gm white petrolatum.

3. Transfer white petrolatum to ointment paper or slab. (Ointment slab is preferred as povidone iodine solution may soak into the paper of the ointment pad.)

4. Make a depression in the white petrolatum, and add a small amount of povidone-iodine solution.

5. Spatulate until evenly mixed.

6. Continue to add small amounts of povidone-iodine solution into a depression in white petrolatum until all is evenly mixed.

7. Check for uniformity of color.

8. Transfer ointment to proper size ointment container being careful to smooth the top of the ointment, and clean the rim and outside of the ointment jar.

9. Apply proper labels.

10. Fill out **Master Formula Sheet.**

11. Clean area, and leave preparation and ingredients for the final check.

PRESCRIPTION 11.2

John Schickel, DO
1801 Lawanna Way
Lansing, MI

<u>Mary Steinhut</u>   **Date**   <u>10-19-06</u>

<u>1276 E. Aurelius Road, Masonville, MI</u>

RX: Menthol   200 mg
       Thymol   200 mg
       Dermabase   60 gm
       Apply to Knee as needed for
       arthritis Pain   John Schickel Do

Sig:

_____   _John Schickel, DO_
Dispense as written   May substitute

Steps:

1. Weigh the menthol and the thymol in separate weighing boats.
2. Mix the two chemicals in a mortar, and triturate with the pestle until the chemicals are liquefied.
3. Place $\frac{1}{3}$ of the Dermabase on an ointment slab or ointment paper.
4. Spatulate with a small amount of the menthol-thymol mixture until evenly mixed.
5. Continue adding the Dermabase and menthol-thymol mixture by geometric dilution and spatulating until all of the chemicals are evenly mixed.
6. Place mixture in a 1-ounce ointment jar.
7. Label with correct information and necessary auxiliary labels.
8. Enter data in **Master Formula Sheet** and leave for final check.

PRESCRIPTION 11.3

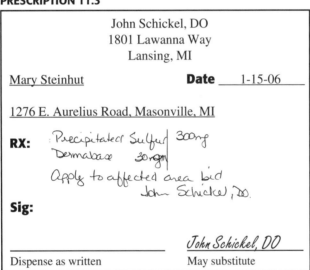

John Schickel, DO
1801 Lawanna Way
Lansing, MI

Mary Steinhut   **Date**   1-15-06

1276 E. Aurelius Road, Masonville, MI

RX: Precipitated Sulfur 300mg
Dermabase   30 gm
Apply to affected area bid
                                      John Schickel, DO.

Sig:

_____   *John Schickel, DO*
Dispense as written   May substitute

Steps:

1. Using the correct weighing technique, weigh the sulfur.
2. Combine sulfur and a few drops of glycerin in glass mortar, and triturate with pestle until it forms a smooth paste.
3. Weigh Dermabase, and transfer to ointment slab or paper.
4. Using geometric dilution, add small amounts of sulfur mixture to small amounts of Dermabase, and spatulate to a smooth cream.
5. Transfer to an appropriate container for dispensing.
6. Label and add any necessary auxiliary labels.
7. Fill out the **Master Formula Sheet** and leave all materials for the final check.

▶ Post-Lab Analysis

1. Describe the appearance of the povidone-iodine-white petrolatum preparation.

   _____

   _____

2. What would you expect to happen if several drops of water were applied to a surface covered with a thin film of the povidone-iodine-white petrolatum ointment?

   _____

3. What is the purpose of the glycerin in the sulfur-Dermabase preparation?

   _____

4. Describe the appearance of the sulfur-Dermabase preparation.

   _____

   _____

5. Would there be a different result if a few drops of water were applied to a thin film of the sulfur-Dermabase preparation compared with what would be observed if a few drops were applied to the product with white petrolatum as the base? Why?

   _____

   _____

6. Calculate the percent of sulfur in the sulfur-Dermabase preparation. _____

MASTER FORMULA SHEET

Compound _____ Quantity _____ Exp Date _____

Student Name _____ Instructor _____ Date _____

INGREDIENT	NDC #	LOT #	QUANTITY	EXP DATE
Notes:				

MASTER FORMULA SHEET

Compound _____ Quantity _____ Exp Date _____

Student Name _____ Instructor _____ Date _____

INGREDIENT	NDC #	LOT #	QUANTITY	EXP DATE
Notes:				

MASTER FORMULA SHEET

Compound _____ Quantity _____ Exp Date _____

Student Name _____ Instructor _____ Date _____

INGREDIENT	NDC #	LOT #	QUANTITY	EXP DATE
Notes:				

MASTER FORMULA SHEET

Compound _____ Quantity _____ Exp Date _____

Student Name _____ Instructor _____ Date _____

INGREDIENT	NDC #	LOT #	QUANTITY	EXP DATE
Notes:				

Lip Balms and Topical Application Sticks

OBJECTIVES

▶ Demonstrate the mixture of two substances that form a eutectic mixture.

▶ Prepare a product with lip balm base to be used as a lubricant and protectant.

▶ Produce a pharmaceutically elegant product in different types of dispensing containers.

▶ Discuss commercial preparations of lip balms and topical application sticks and their uses.

Lip balms can be primarily used for lubrication or they may contain cooling ingredients such as menthol, an antibiotic to prevent infection, an antiviral to alleviate the discomfort of cold sores, a topical anesthetic, or a combination of several of these agents. Likewise larger stick applications can be formulated to be applied to other parts of the body. The shape of the medication stick can be adapted to the site of application. These products are very portable and convenient, eliminating the need to apply the product with the hands.

▶ Pre-Lab Questions

1. What type of agents could be added to a commercial lip balm formulation to increase the hardness of the product and make it suitable for a larger topical application stick?

   _____

2. Why would the addition of zinc oxide to an emollient stick formulation make it suitable for a hot, sunny day at the beach?

   _____

   _____

3. How would you determine the expiration date for a lip balm or applicator stick formulation?

   _____

   _____

   _____

4. List the therapeutic use for the following lip balm and medication stick formulations:

   Carmex _____

   Blistex Ultra Protection Stick _____

   Chap Stick Medicated Stick _____

   Cortaid Maximum Strength Faststick _____

   Palmer's Cocoa Butter Stick _____

   Ben-Gay Icy Chill Stick _____

▶ Lab Exercises

Prepare the compound indicated in the prescription, following the instructions detailed in the Steps.

Peter James, MD
6417 Lily Drive, Fairview, WI 65034
Phone: 642-562-1943

Name: Sally Flowers   **Date:** 01-15-06

Address: 7560 West Grant Boulevard, Fairview, WI 65033

RX: Menthol   1%
Thymol   1%
Lip Balm Base   qs to make lip
balm stick (15gm)
Sig: Apply to sore on lip prn until
gone.

Peter James, MD

_____   _____
Dispense as written   May substitute

Steps:

1. Weigh 150 mg of menthol crystals in a weighing boat and set aside.

2. Weigh 150 mg of thymol crystals and set aside.

3. Weigh 15 grams of lip balm base.

4. Mix the menthol and thymol in a glass beaker with a glass stirring rod until they liquefy.

5. Prepare a hot water bath by pouring hot water in a large beaker.

6. Place the lip balm base in the beaker with the liquefied eutectic mixture.

7. Place the beaker with the lip balm mixture in the larger beaker that has been prepared with hot water.

8. Stir the mixture with a glass stirring rod until it is completely liquefied and clear.

9. Using care with the hot materials, pour the mixture into a lip balm applicator.

10. As the mixture begins to solidify in the applicator, a small depression will form in the center. Add more lip balm mixture to fill in this depression.

11. Pour the remaining lip balm mixture into a small ointment jar.

12. Allow mixture to solidify in both containers.

13. Prepare the **Master Formula Sheet.**

14. Prepare and apply labels to each container.

15. Place materials in the appropriate place for a final check.

▶ Post-Lab Analysis

1. What purpose would the menthol and thymol serve in this formulation?

   _____

   _____

2. What storage requirements would be appropriate for this formulation?

   _____

   _____

3. What would be the therapeutic use of a lip balm formulation containing acyclovir?

   _____

4. How would the consistency of the formulation be altered if a wax was added to the formula?

   _____

   _____

5. What would be a possible therapeutic use for a larger medication stick made with acyclovir and a wax content to provide desired consistency?

   _____

MASTER FORMULA SHEET

Compound ———————————— Quantity ———— Exp Date ————

Student Name ———————— Instructor ———————— Date ————

INGREDIENT	NDC #	LOT #	QUANTITY	EXP DATE
Notes:				

MASTER FORMULA SHEET

Compound ———————————— Quantity ———— Exp Date ————

Student Name ———————— Instructor ———————— Date ————

INGREDIENT	NDC #	LOT #	QUANTITY	EXP DATE
Notes:				

Suppositories

TERMS

Rectal

Urethral

Palliative

Protectant

Systemic

Vaginal

Density factor

Displacement

EQUIPMENT AND INGREDIENTS

Prescription balance

Mortar/pestle

Spatula

Cocoa butter

Hot plate

Beaker

Ibuprofen powder

White filter paper

Disposable suppository molds

Foil wrappers

Prescription vials

Vegetable spray

OBJECTIVES

▶ Discuss the advantages of suppositories as a dosage form.

▶ List the various routes of administration that can accommodate a suppository dosage form.

▶ Prepare a suppository formulation using disposable suppository molds.

▶ Demonstrate preparation of hand-rolled cocoa butter base suppositories.

▶ List factors that must be considered when preparing a suppository dosage form.

▶ Pre-Lab Questions

1. List two conditions where the use of a suppository formulation would be superior to an oral dosage form.

   _____

   _____

2. Describe a specific condition in which each of the following routes of suppository administration would be beneficial.

   Vaginal_____

   Rectal_____

   Urethral_____

3. What storage instructions should be placed on the label of a compounded suppository?

   _____

4. List approximate weights for the following suppository dosage forms:

   Adult Rectal _____

   Vaginal _____

   Pediatric Rectal _____

   Male Urethral _____

   Female Urethral _____

5. List 6 steps for proper insertion of a rectal suppository in an adult.

   _____

   _____

   _____

   _____

   _____

   _____

6. Why does the dose of the drug need to be more accurately calculated using the density factor if the formulation is intended for its systemic effect instead of the topical effect?

   _____

   _____

   _____

7. The density factor of ibuprofen powder is 1.1 g. This means that 1 gram of ibuprofen will displace 1.1 grams of cocoa butter. Since this suppository will be used for the systemic effect of ibuprofen, it is important to consider the displacement effect when calculating the amounts of cocoa butter and ibuprofen needed to compound the suppositories.

   If a suppository mold produces a suppository with an average weight of 1.9 g, calculate the amounts of ibuprofen powder and cocoa butter needed to compound a prescription for six suppositories. Make enough for two extra suppositories. Use the following steps to perform these calculations.

Amount of ibuprofen needed for 8 suppositories each containing 200 mg

_____ (a)

$$\frac{1.1 \text{ g of ibuprofen}}{1\text{g of cocoa butter}} = \frac{\text{total g of ibuprofen needed (a)}}{\text{X (number of grams of cocoa butter)}} = \begin{array}{l}\text{grams of cocoa}\\\text{butter displaced}\\\text{by ibuprofen (c)}\end{array}$$

Total weight of 8 suppositories (b) − displacement factor (c) = $\begin{array}{l}\text{grams of cocoa}\\\text{butter needed for}\\\text{8 suppositories}\end{array}$

▶ Lab Exercises

Using the calculations in question 7 of the Pre-Lab Questions, prepare the ibuprofen suppositories in the following prescription.

Jeffery Raker, MD
5067 Winston Drive, Baltimore, MD 56772
546-355-7743

Name: Mary Sullivan   **Date:** 04-25-06

Address: 2403 East Haverford, Baltimore, MD 56832

RX:

Ibuprofen 200 mg
Cocoa butter qs
make and dispense 6 suppositories

Sig: insert 1 suppository q 4h prn
arthritis pain

_____   *Jeffery Raker, MD*
Dispense as written   May substitute

Steps:

▶ Weigh the calculated amount of ibuprofen powder, adding a little extra for any loss that may occur during trituration and transfer.

▶ Triturate the ibuprofen with a mortar and pestle until a fine powder is produced to facilitate solution in the warm cocoa butter.

▶ Weigh the amount of the finely powdered ibuprofen and set aside.

▶ Weigh the calculated amount of cocoa butter and grate it into small pieces.

▶ Prepare the suppository molds by spraying lightly with vegetable spray.

▶ Prepare a warm water bath around 55 degrees centigrade.

▶ Warm a small portion of the cocoa butter until just melted and add the ibuprofen.

▶ Stir until dissolved and continue adding the cocoa butter until all is melted.

▶ Be careful to keep the water bath temperature from overheating.

▶ Pour the mixture into the suppository mold using all the mixture for the eight suppositories. Molds may need to be overfilled slightly because the mixture will contract as it cools.

▶ Leave the suppositories at room temperature until they have hardened completely.

▶ After they have hardened, place in refrigerator for 30 minutes.

▶ Trim any excess from the top of the suppositories and clean mold.

▶ Place disposable mold with suppositories in a container suitable for dispensing.

▶ Apply label with appropriate directions for storage and use.

▶ Document procedure on a **Master Formula Sheet** and leave with paperwork for final check.

Using the same calculations as for the earlier prescription, prepare the suppositories by the hand-rolled method.

Steps:

- ▶ Weigh the powdered ibuprofen and triturate to a fine powder.
- ▶ Weigh the cocoa butter and shave into small pieces if necessary.
- ▶ Add a small amount of cocoa butter to the ibuprofen in the mortar and triturate until well mixed.
- ▶ Continue to add small amounts of cocoa butter, using geometric dilution and trituration until all has been added.
- ▶ Mix until a plastic mass has been formed.
- ▶ Using disposable gloves, transfer the mass to a piece of white filter paper.
- ▶ Knead the mixture until a uniform mass is formed.
- ▶ Place on an ointment slab and roll into an 8-inch cylinder.
- ▶ Using a metal spatula, divide the roll into eight equal pieces.
- ▶ Shape each suppository with a pointed end and weigh each piece.
- ▶ Suppository should weigh 2 grams each within a margin of error of 5% or less.
- ▶ Trim any excess with a razor blade and wrap each suppository in foil.
- ▶ Place in an appropriate container for dispensing and prepare label.
- ▶ Document procedure on a **Master Formula Sheet** and leave all materials for final check.

▶ Post-Lab Analysis

1. Compare the two suppository formulations for the following factors:

   Ease of preparation_____

   _____

   Time required_____

   _____

   Pharmaceutical elegance_____

   _____

2. If the patient, Mary Sullivan, was an 8-year-old girl weighing 50 pounds, discuss the appropriateness of the dose and size of the suppository formulation.

   _____

3. Why would a drug that is highly metabolized by the first-pass effect in the liver perform better when administered in a suppository formulation?

_____

_____

4. Acetaminophen 120-mg rectal suppositories are available commercially, but pharmacist Smith is able to make these suppositories in his compounding pharmacy and market them to physicians in the area. Discuss the legality of this.

_____

_____

_____

5. List two advantages of disposable suppository molds over nondisposable molds.

_____

_____

6. Using reference materials, provide an example of a commercial suppository preparation with each of the following therapeutic uses:

Systemic antiemetic _____

Topical anti-inflammatory _____

Systemic analgesic _____

Local laxative _____

Vaginal antifungal _____

Rectal lubricant _____

MASTER FORMULA SHEET

Compound _____ Quantity _____ Exp Date _____

Student Name _____ Instructor _____ Date _____

INGREDIENT	NDC #	LOT #	QUANTITY	EXP DATE
Notes:				

MASTER FORMULA SHEET

Compound _____ Quantity _____ Exp Date _____

Student Name _____ Instructor _____ Date _____

INGREDIENT	NDC #	LOT #	QUANTITY	EXP DATE
Notes:				

Lozenges

OBJECTIVES

▶ List the reasons for compounding medications in a lozenge formulation.

▶ Demonstrate the ability to compound a hand-rolled lozenge formulation.

▶ Use a mold to prepare a hard lozenge base.

▶ Prepare a gummy gel formulation for administering medications.

The lozenge dosage form provides an administration route that is pleasant and palatable. Some benefits of lozenges are that they can soothe an irritated throat, they offer topical application of agents used for fungal and bacterial infections of the oral cavity, and they are an alternative oral dosage form for patients who have difficulty swallowing other oral solids.

▶ Pre-Lab Questions

1. What special caution should be issued to parents of small children when dispensing medications in a gummy bear base or sweet-tasting lozenge?

   _____

2. Discuss the advantage of using a lozenge formulation for an antifungal agent to treat thrush in a young child.

   _____

   _____

3. Why would a candy-making cookbook be helpful when researching formulas for hard lozenges?

   _____

   _____

4. There is a commercial sugar-based lozenge on a stick formulation of fentanyl (brand name: Actiq). Discuss the differences between this product and the fentanyl formulation (Oralet), including flavor, onset, duration, and specific indications.

   _____

   _____

   _____

   _____

5. Name three over-the-counter lozenge formulations and give their uses.

   _____

   _____

   _____

▶ Lab Exercises

Hand-Rolled Lozenges

Follow the procedure detailed in the Steps for Prescription 14.1.

PRESCRIPTION 14.1

Michael Mordo, M.D.
3798 Golden Rodeo Drive
Palo Alto, CO 80634

Name: Marcia Marathon   **Date:** 4-25-06

1223 Dallas Drive, Hoboken, IL 46304

RX:
Clotrimazol 100mg
Acacia 0.7g
Powdered sugar 10g
Purified water qs
Cherry flavor 5 drops
Red food coloring 5 drops
Dispense 10 lozenges containing 10mg each of active ingredient

Sig: Dissolve one lozenge in mouth Bid x 5 days.

Michael Mordo, MD

Dispense as written   May substitute

Steps:

1. Calculate weight of ingredients needed to make the required 10 lozenges plus 2 extra.

2. 10 mg of clotrimazole × 12 lozenges = 120 mg clotrimazole

   11.18 g powdered sugar

   0.7 g of acacia

   Total weight of ingredients = 12 g/12 lozenges = 1 g/lozenge

3. Weigh each of the ingredients in a weighing boat.

4. Place acacia in a glass mortar and add 2 ml of water, 5 drops of cherry flavor, and 5 drops of red food coloring.

5. Triturate mixture to form a mucilage.

6. Place clotrimazole and powdered sugar in a flour sifter and sift powders onto an ointment pad.

7. Gradually add powdered sugar/clotrimazole mix to acacia mucilage in mortar.

8. Triturate until evenly mixed and dough-like.

9. Wearing gloves, roll mass into a cylinder and measure with ruler.

10. Cut into 12 even pieces.

11. Weigh finished lozenges. Each should weigh approximately 1 g.

12. Calculate the % variation from 1 g.

13. Wrap each lozenge in foil wrapper.

14. Package the 10 lozenges that are closest to 1 g in weight in an appropriate container and label.

15. Fill out formula log and leave materials and paperwork for final check.

Molded "Gummy Gel" Lozenges

Follow the procedure detailed in the Steps for Prescription 14.2.

PRESCRIPTION 14.2

Michael Mordo, MD
3798 Golden Rodeo Drive
Palo Alto, CO 80634

Name: Marcia Marathon   **Date:** 04-25-06

1223 Dallas Drive, Hoboken, IL 46304

RX: Clotrimazole 100mg
Flavor and color additives as needed
Lozibase   qs

Dispense 10 lozenges containing 10mg each
of active ingredient
Sig: Dissolve one lozenge in mouth Bid x 5 days

Refill 0 1 2 3

_____   *Michael Mordo, MD*_____

Dispense as written   May substitute

Steps:

1. Prepare adequate mixture for two extra lozenges.
2. 10 mg clotrimazole $\times$ 12 lozenges = 120 mg clotrimazole
3. Weigh clotrimazole in weighing boat and set aside.
4. Weigh empty mold and spray lightly with vegetable spray.
5. Melt lozi-base in water bath.
6. Add 5 drops of yellow food coloring and 5 drops of lemon flavoring.
7. Fill 12 slots in mold with flavored lozi-base.
8. Weigh filled mold and remove 120 mg of base.
9. Return lozi-base remaining in mold to water bath.
10. Add clotrimazole powder to mold and stir until dissolved.
11. Pour mixture into 12 slots of mold and allow to harden.
12. Weigh filled mold to check for accuracy.
13. When solidified, remove two extra lozenges from mold.
14. Clean mold with soft tissue.
15. Prepare appropriate labeling, fill out **Master Formula Sheet**, and leave paperwork with calculations for final check.

Hard Candy Molded Lozenges

Follow the preparation and procedure detailed in the Steps for Prescription 14.3.

PRESCRIPTION 14.3

Michael Mordo, MD
3798 Golden Rodeo Drive
Palo Alto, CO 80634

Name: Marcia Marathon   **Date:** 04-25-06

1223 Dallas Drive, Hoboken, IL 46304

RX:

Ibuprofen 200mg

Prepare 10 lozenges in a hard candy base each containing 200mg Ibuprofen

Sig: Dissolve one lozenge in mouth qid

Refill 0 1 2 3

_____   *Michael Mordo, MD*
Dispense as written   May substitute

Preparation: Prepare enough hard candy mixture for the entire class using the following proportions as a guideline.

Dextrose	70 g
Light Corn syrup	40 g
Distilled water	20 ml
Flavoring	0.5 ml
Coloring	4–5 drops
Ibuprofen	_____

Steps:

1. Prepare 10 ml of hard candy mixture for each lozenge.
2. Mix dextrose, corn syrup, and water in a beaker and place in a water bath on a hot plate.
3. Heat and stir until the dextrose is dissolved and temperature of mixture is 154 degrees centigrade on candy thermometer.
4. Remove from heat and stir in flavoring and coloring.
5. Measure 100 ml of liquid candy mixture into small beaker and add 2 grams of ibuprofen powder.
6. Lightly spray insides of 10 dosing cups and divide mixture evenly in the 10 cups using the measuring guidelines on the cup to assure accuracy.
7. Allow to harden and individually wrap in plastic wrap.
8. Document ingredients and expiration date on **Master Formula Sheet**.
9. Prepare label and leave product and paperwork for the final check.

▶ Post-Lab Analysis

1. Compare the three lozenge formulation in terms of the following factors:

   a. Ease of preparation:_____

   _____

   _____

   b. Pharmaceutical elegance of final product:_____

   _____

   _____

2. What added benefit may be derived from administering ibuprofen in a lozenge form to treat throat pain?

_____

_____

3. Discuss the importance of solubility and temperature stability when preparing a hard candy formulation.

_____

_____

_____

4. Name two age categories of patients who would benefit from medications delivered in a lozenge form.

   a. _____

   b. _____

5. How would you determine the expiration dates for the lozenges prepared in this exercise?

_____

_____

MASTER FORMULA SHEET

Compound _____ Quantity _____ Exp Date _____

Student Name _____ Instructor _____ Date _____

INGREDIENT	NDC #	LOT #	QUANTITY	EXP DATE
Notes:				

MASTER FORMULA SHEET

Compound _____ Quantity _____ Exp Date _____

Student Name _____ Instructor _____ Date _____

INGREDIENT	NDC #	LOT #	QUANTITY	EXP DATE
Notes:				

MASTER FORMULA SHEET

Compound _____ Quantity _____ Exp Date _____

Student Name _____ Instructor _____ Date _____

INGREDIENT	NDC #	LOT #	QUANTITY	EXP DATE
Notes:				

MASTER FORMULA SHEET

Compound _____ Quantity _____ Exp Date _____

Student Name _____ Instructor _____ Date _____

INGREDIENT	NDC #	LOT #	QUANTITY	EXP DATE
Notes:				

Veterinary Compounds

OBJECTIVES

▶ Compound a topical ointment suitable for skin disorders of animals.

▶ Prepare a palatable suspension for an animal from a tablet or capsule dosage form.

▶ Demonstrate appropriate record keeping for veterinary prescriptions.

▶ Explain prescribing authority for a veterinarian.

Veterinary compounding provides a service for pet owners to receive a custom product prescribed by the personal veterinarian of the pet. Changing the dosage form and adding flavorings to make the drug more palatable for the animal will facilitate administration of the product.

▶ Pre-Lab Questions

1. When might it be appropriate to fill a prescription for a patient named "Arthur" White that was written by a veterinarian?

_____

_____

2. What do the letters DVM indicate?

_____

3. What notation would you make on the prescription for the patient "Arthur" White if the prescription was for Jim White's German Shepherd?

_____

_____

4. What types of medications is a DVM allowed to prescribe?

_____

_____

5. What requirements exist for the prescribing of controlled drugs by a DVM?

_____

_____

▶ Lab Exercises

Prepare the two following prescriptions using the directions detailed in the Steps after each prescription.

PRESCRIPTION 15.1

James Harreot, DVM
1203 Hidden Valley Road, Indianapolis, IN 46883

Name: Canine "Arthur" White   **Date** 7/5/05

642 South Groge Street, Avon, Indiana 46732

RX: SULFUR POWDER   10%
                 SALICYLIC ACID   5%

          QS TO 60g WITH WHITE PETROLATUM.

Sig: APPLY TO AREAS OF SKIN AFFECTED BY MANGE BID

                                        James Harreot, DVM
_____
Dispense as written   May substitute

Steps:

1. Calculate the amount of sulfur powder needed for the preparation. Label and circle answer.
2. Weigh the sulfur and set aside in a weighing boat
3. Calculate the amount of salicylic acid needed. Label and circle answer.
4. Weigh the salicylic acid in a weighing boat and set aside.
5. Add a small amount of alcohol to the salicylic acid and stir until dissolved.
6. Add a small amount of glycerin to sulfur powder and form a smooth paste.
7. Calculate the amount of petrolatum needed by subtracting the combined weights of the sulfur and the salicylic acid from 60 g.
8. Weigh the correct amount of white petrolatum and place on an ointment slab or paper.
9. Divide the petrolatum approximately in half on the paper.
10. Using geometric dilution and a spatula, begin mixing small portions of the petrolatum with small amounts of sulfur mixture until all is added.
11. Using geometric dilution and a spatula, begin adding salicylic acid mixture to small amounts of white petrolatum until all is mixed.
12. Continuing with geometric dilution, begin spatulating small amount of the sulfur-white petrolatum mixture with small amounts of the salicylic acid-white petrolatum mixture.
13. Continue spatulation until the mixture is well mixed and uniform in color.

14. Dispense in an ointment jar.
15. Record ingredients and compounding techniques on a **Master Formula Sheet**.
16. Prepare a prescription label and apply auxiliary labels.
17. Place in the designated place for final check.

PRESCRIPTION 15.2

James Harreot, DVM
1203 Hidden Valley Road, Indianapolis, IN 46883

Name: Feline "Sassy" White   **Date** 7/5/05

642 South Groge Street, Avon, IN 46732

RX: FUROSEMIDE SUSPENSION   1 mg/ml

Quantity: 60 ml

Sig: GIVE 3 cc each day IN THE MORNING. MAY ADD TO SMALL AMOUNT
OF TUNA OR USE ORAL SYRINGE TO ADMINISTER

James Harreot, DVM

Dispense as written   May substitute

Steps:

1. Calculate the number of 20-mg furosemide tablets needed for this compound.
2. Place tablets in mortar and triturate until reduced to a fine powder.
3. Add small amount of Ora Plus and triturate until a smooth paste is formed.
4. Add 20 ml more of Ora Plus and mix well.
5. Add 10 cc of bacon flavoring and mix well.
6. Pour into appropriate size graduate and qs to 60 ml.
7. Mix well and pour into 60-ml prescription bottle.
8. Document ingredients and technique on **Master Formula Sheet.**
9. Prepare label and auxiliary labels.
10. Place product and paperwork on table for final check.

NOTE - Veterinary prescriptions require the following statement to be on the label: "Caution: Federal law restricts this drug for use by or on the order of a licensed Veterinarian."

▶ Post-Lab Analysis

1. Define mange.

   _____

   _____

2. Explain possible therapeutic uses of each of the ingredients in the ointment preparation for the canine.

   Sulfur_____

   Salicylic Acid _____

   White Petrolatum_____

3. What administration device needs to be included with the prescription for the feline?

   _____

4. What information is required to be on a prescription for a controlled drug written for an animal by a veterinarian?

   _____

   _____

   _____

   _____

MASTER FORMULA SHEET

Compound _____ Quantity _____ Exp Date _____

Student Name _____ Instructor _____ Date _____

INGREDIENT	NDC #	LOT #	QUANTITY	EXP DATE
Notes:				

MASTER FORMULA SHEET

Compound _____ Quantity _____ Exp Date _____

Student Name _____ Instructor _____ Date _____

INGREDIENT	NDC #	LOT #	QUANTITY	EXP DATE
Notes:				

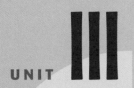

UNIT **III**

Intravenous Admixtures

CHAPTER 16

Large-Volume Parenterals

TERMS

Large-volume parenteral
LVP
Aseptic technique
Sterility
Laminar airflow workbench
LAFW
HEPA filter
Risk levels
Compatibility
D5W
NSS
Zone of turbulence

EQUIPMENT

1 L bag D5W
1 L Bag NS
Alcohol
Alcohol swabs
Horizontal laminar flow workbench
Syringes
Needles
Hand-washing supplies
Gloves and gowns
Additive vials
Hair coverings
Face masks

OBJECTIVES

▶ Discuss the uses of single-use large-volume parenterals.

▶ List disadvantages of parenteral therapy.

▶ Demonstrate proper hand-washing and gowning techniques.

▶ Effectively clean and prepare the laminar flow hood.

▶ Demonstrate appropriate aseptic technique for injecting an additive into a large-volume bag.

Large-volume parenterals are important tools in maintenance therapy for daily body fluids, in replacement therapy for fluid losses, and for restoring fluids during times of continuing fluid loss. In addition to replacing fluid loss and maintaining fluid balance, maintenance IV therapy can provide nutrients and electrolytes to meet the daily needs of the patient. Maintaining the appropriate balance may require the addition, under aseptic conditions, of electrolytes, vitamins, or other agents as ordered by the prescriber. An extensive discussion of risk levels, aseptic technique, and the new regulations outlined by USP 797 should precede this exercise. Exercises in this book are considered to be Risk Level 1 unless otherwise stated by the instructor.

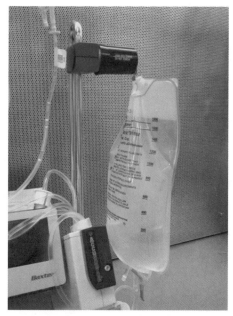

Large volume parenteral solution packaged in pliable plastic. (Courtesy of Ms. Amy Schuppert Smith.)

▶ Pre-Lab Questions

1. List five reasons for using parenteral therapy.

_____

_____

_____

_____

_____

2. List three disadvantages of the parenteral route of administration.

_____

_____

_____

3. Discuss the HEPA filter. What do the letters stand for, and what is the filtering capacity of a HEPA filter?

_____

_____

_____

4. Discuss the appropriate method for cleaning a laminar flow hood in preparation for IV admixture.

_____

_____

_____

5. Describe the steps for hand-washing in preparation for IV admixture.

_____

_____

_____

6. Describe the appropriate method for preparing vials before entering with a needle.

_____

_____

7. List the appropriate dress requirements for preparing IV products classified as Risk Level 1.

_____

_____

_____

_____

▶ Lab Exercises

Prepare the following large-volume IV admixtures using proper hand-washing and gowning techniques according to the protocol established by the instructor for Risk Level 1 and strict aseptic technique. Follow the technique shown in the diagrams for entering vials and IV bag ports and the procedure outlined in the Steps to prepare IV.

Medication Order 16.1

Date/Time _____   Medication Orders _____

IVF: _NS + 100 mEq ammonium chloride_

                             infuse @ 125 cc/hr

Nursing Notes: _Monitor levels of serum bicarbonate_

                  Mary Dearing, MD

Medical Orders   **Patient Information**
                      John Jacobs 8/29/60   44 yo male

Pharmacy Copy

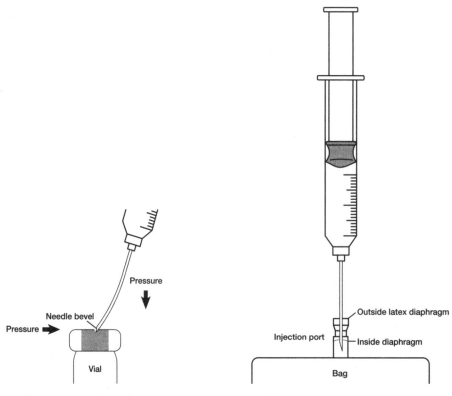

Needle penetration of a vial to prevent coring.   *Needle penetration of an IV injection port.*

Steps:

1. Check the medication order for reasonable dose, infusion rate, concentration of solution, and route of administration

2. Check for stability and compatibility of solution

3. Prepare appropriate IV labels.

4. Remove jewelry and wash, gown, and glove according to protocol.

5. Use appropriate technique for cleaning LAFW with 70% isopropyl alcohol.

6. Select an appropriate size syringe and needle.

7. Determine the correct amount of ammonium chloride needed if the vial on hand contains 5 mEq/ml and contains 20 ml. _____

8. Add the appropriate amount of air to the ammonium chloride vial.

9. Using aseptic technique to draw up the appropriate amount of ammonium chloride into the syringe.

10. Be certain when entering the injection port of the IV bag that the needle penetrates both diaphragms of the port and does not puncture the bag or the side of the port.

11. Discard the trash, and apply the label to the IV bag

12. Leave the bottle and syringe along with the paperwork for the final check.

Demonstrate the ability to follow a step-by-step procedure using correct aseptic technique to produce the following IV admixture. Note the procedural steps in the space allowed in the Post-Lab Analysis.

Medication Order 16.2

Date/Time _____	Medication Orders _____
IVF:	D5W 1L add 20 meq magnesium sulfate infuse @ 125 cc/hour
Nursing Notes:	Continue for 3 days *Mary Denning, MD*
Medical Orders	**Patient Information** Sally Fairchild 57 yo female
Pharmacy Copy	

▶ Post-Lab Analysis

1. List the steps used in the preparation of the IV admixture of D5W/magnesium sulfate. If the magnesium sulfate on hand is 4 mEq/ml, tell how many ml of magnesium sulfate will be added.

_____

_____

_____

_____

_____

_____

_____

2. Discuss the correct procedure for extracting fluid from a sealed vial. Include equalization of air pressure and appropriate technique for entering a sealed vial with a needle.

_____

_____

_____

3. Describe the correct procedure for entering an IV port with a needle.

_____

_____

_____

4. Explain the zone of turbulence and the need to work 6 inches inside the hood.

_____

_____

_____

IV Piggybacks and Small-Volume Parenterals

OBJECTIVES

▶ Discuss the difference between a large-volume parenteral and small-volume parenteral.

▶ Describe how an IV piggyback is used in conjunction with a large-volume parenteral.

▶ Demonstrate reconstitution of sterile powders for addition to an IV piggyback.

▶ Demonstrate proper technique for withdrawing medication from an ampule

▶ Demonstrate proficiency in addition of medications to a small-volume parenteral bag.

Agents manufactured for IV infusion are available in several forms of sterile packaging. Proper manipulation of these devices is essential to the maintenance of a sterile product suitable for IV administration to the patient.

▶ Pre-Lab Questions

1. Patient Jean Jones has a standing order for 1000 ml of D5W to infuse at 125 cc/hr for fluid maintenance. Elevated temperature and bronchial congestion indicate a developing infection, so her physician sends an order to the pharmacy for 1 g of Rocephin to be infused IV bid. Answer the following questions about this scenario.

   a. Describe the type of small-volume parenteral you would prepare to infuse this with in conjunction with the maintenance large-volume parenteral.

   _____

   b. If you had available a 2-g vial of Rocephin powder for reconstitution, how much sterile water for injection should be added to produce a final volume of 8 ml? (Check reference book, package insert, or Rocephin bottle.)

   _____

   c. What is the volume of the powder displacement?

   _____

   d. What is the mg/ml strength of the Rocephin solution after reconstitution?

   _____

   e. Describe the small-volume IV bag(s) you would choose to mix this piggyback order.

   _____

   f. When preparing the IV bags for one 24-hour period, how many bags will you prepare?

   _____

   g. How many ml of the reconstituted Rocephin solution will you add to each bag?

   _____

   h. What auxiliary labels would you apply to the Rocephin bags?

   _____

2. Describe the procedure for opening a sealed glass ampule.

   _____

   _____

   _____

   _____

3. Describe the procedure for withdrawing medication from an ampule using a filter straw or a filter needle.

_____

_____

_____

_____

_____

▶ Lab Exercises

Prepare a 24-hour supply of the IV medications in the following medication orders.

Medication Order 17.1

Date/Time 05-06-06   Medication Orders _____

D5W/KCl 10 meq/L infuse at 125ml/h
Timentin 3.1g IVPB q4h
                  J Manning MD

Medical Orders

Patient Information
Sandra Sanders 57 yo female

Pharmacy Copy

How many 1-L bags of D5W/KCl 10 will be needed for 1 day? _____

What size and type of IVPB bag will you use for the Timentin? _____

How many IVPB bags will be needed for a 24-hour supply? _____

How many 3.1-g vials of Timentin will be needed? _____

Steps:

1. Follow protocol for hand-washing and gowning.
2. Clean IV hood.
3. Gather ingredients and arrange appropriately in hood.
4. Wipe all ports with alcohol.
5. Using aseptic technique, add 13 ml of SWI to each Timentin sterile powder vial.
6. Shake well until powder is dissolved.
7. Each 5 ml of the reconstituted Timentin contains 1 g of Timentin.
8. Add 15 ml of Timentin solution to each of the IVPB bags.
9. Rotate bags to evenly distribute drug.
10. Cover IV port of each bag with an IV seal.
11. Inspect each bag for any particulate matter.
12. Label each bag appropriately and leave with paperwork, vials, and syringes used for final check.
13. Discard unused materials not needed for the final check.
14. Clean the hood.

Medication Order 17.2

Date/Time 05-03-06   Medication Orders _____

Lasix 40mg / D5W 100ml

Infuse over 30 minutes once daily

M Amado M D

Medical Orders

Patient Information
Sandra Smithson   45 yo female

Pharmacy Copy

Steps:

1. Use 4-ml ampule of Lasix 10 mg/ml and 100-ml minibag of D5W.

2. Remove jewelry, and wash and gown according to protocol.

3. Clean the LAFW with 70% alcohol using the side to side, back to front technique.

4. Assemble all materials in hood: 4-ml Lasix ampule, D5W 100-ml minibag, 5-ml syringe, needle, and filter straw.

5. Wipe ampule and minibag port with alcohol.

6. To open the ampule, wrap an alcohol pad around the neck of the ampule. Holding the ampule firmly, snap the top off the ampule with the thumb. (If the ampule top does not snap easily, rotate the ampule slightly and apply pressure again.)

7. Attach a filter straw or filter needle to the syringe and withdraw 4 ml of fluid from the ampule.

8. Holding the syringe upright to prevent loss of fluid, remove the filter straw or filter needle and attach a sterile needle to the syringe.

9. Inject the Lasix into the port of the minibag.

10. Rotate bag to evenly distribute drug.

11. Visually inspect fluid in bag for any particulate matter.

12. Apply seal to the port.

13. Apply label, expiration date, and auxiliary labels to the bag, discard unneeded materials, and leave the product for the final check.

14. Clean hood with alcohol to wipe any spills.

▶ Post-Lab Analysis

1. In the medication order for Timentin 3.1 g, what was the approximate volume of the liquid Timentin solution in each vial after reconstitution?

_____

2. What was the amount of powder displacement in the above question?

_____

3. Name the two ingredients in Timentin.

_____

4. What is the therapeutic purpose of clavulanate?

_____

5. What is the general antibiotic class of ticarcillin?

_____

_____

6. Sandra Smithson developed a high fever indicating an infection. Dr. Amado ordered the addition of Amikacin 500 mg bid infused over 30 minutes to her medication regimen. What toxic effects would be a concern when using Lasix and Amikacin together?

_____

7. What precautions should be taken to monitor for the adverse effects in question 6?

_____

_____

8. On delivering the IV bags to the patient, floor you overheard the nurses speaking in an unusually loud voice to Sandra Smithson. What question would you want to ask to determine if her hearing impairment was caused by the concomitant administration of Lasix and Amikacin?

_____

_____

Total Parenteral Nutrition

OBJECTIVES

▶ Discuss conditions that may necessitate total parenteral nutrition.

▶ List the usual base components and the function of each in a TPN.

▶ List common additives used in TPNs.

▶ Manually prepare a TPN mixture using aseptic technique in a laboratory.

▶ Discuss the use of automatic compounding devices for preparing a TPN.

Total parenteral nutrition is a vital part of therapy for patients unable to receive adequate nutrition through the enteral route. Most hospital facilities have commercial automated compounding equipment to facilitate this labor-intensive procedure. Smaller home-infusion pharmacies may not have the volume of TPN orders to make the purchase of automated compounders cost-effective. This exercise will provide hands-on experience in manual compounding of a TPN admixture and a discussion of basic procedures for the use of an automated system.

▶ Pre-Lab Questions

1. List three patient situations where total parenteral nutrition would be required.

   _____

   _____

   _____

2. What are three disadvantages of total parenteral nutrition?

   _____

   _____

   _____

3. List the base components of a TPN and their purpose.

   _____

   _____

   _____

4. List the common electrolytes often included in a TPN.

   _____

   _____

   _____

5. Discuss the difference between the administration of a PPN and a TPN.

   _____

   _____

6. What is the time frame for beginning infusion of a TPN bag that has been stored at room temperature?

_____

7. Why is warming of a TPN bag a cause for concern?

_____

8. Why is the order of addition of ingredients in a TPN important?

_____

9. What will happen if potassium phosphate is added to the TPN bag after the addition of calcium gluconate?

_____

_____

▶ Lab Exercise

Prepare the following TPN order using the manual fill gravity method of admixture.

Patient Name: *GD*	Location: *TLC-480*		Medical Record # *200440*

Dosing Weight: 80 kg   Administration Date/Time: *00/01/00 @ 1600*

Expiration Date/Time: *00/02/00 @ 1600*   Bag ID #: *001*

Infusion Volume Ordered: *2400 mL*   Infusion Rate: *100 mL/hr*

Base Components	Concentration	Dose Ordered	Volume (mL)
Protein	Travasol 10%	120 g	1200
Dextrose	D70W	346	494
Fat Emulsion	20%	55	275

Additives	Concentration	Dose Ordered	Volume (mL)
Sodium Phosphate	3 mmol P/mL	30 mEq	10
	4 mEq Na/mL		
Sodium Chloride	4 mEq/mL	110 mEq	27.5
Potassium Acetate	2 mEq/mL	80 mEq	40
Magnesium Sulfate	4 mEq/mL	24 mEq	6
Calcium Gluconate	0.45 mEq/mL	10 mEq	22.2
Adult Multivitamins	———	10 mL	10
Trace Elements	———	3 mL	3
Ranitidine	25 mg/mL	150 mg	6

Additives per ion:	
Na	150 mEq
K	80 mEq
Mg	24 mEq
Ca	10 mEq
Ac	80 mEq
Cl	110 mEq
P	30 mmol

Calculate the amount of SWI needed to bring the total volume of the TPN to the 2400 ml per day ordered by adding the volume of all other additives and subtracting the total from 2400 ml: _____.

Additive calculations have been completed by the pharmacist. The technician should double check each vial to be certain the concentration is as stated in the formula and the pharmacist's calculations are correct.

Steps:

1. Use hand-washing procedure and don appropriate garb.

2. Clean the LAFW with 70% alcohol (or agent approved by site) using front to back, side to side technique.

3. Gather all needed materials and place appropriately in the hood with special attention to the zone of turbulence and ability to work without blocking air flow. At this time, perform another check to ascertain that each vial is the correct drug and concentration.

4. Check all expiration dates before proceeding.

5. Use the gravity method to hang each of the base components and add them to the empty large-volume sterile IV bag in the order listed in the IV order form.

6. Site protocol may require a pharmacist check before adding electrolytes.

7. Begin adding the additives, using aseptic technique. Be sure that the phosphate is the first electrolyte added and that calcium is the last electrolyte to be added to the admixture.

8. Any additive vials that may be re-used must be labeled with the date, the time it was first opened, and the initials of the person opening it.

9. Apply a seal to the ports of the TPN bag and remove it to the area where the label can be applied.

10. Leave labeled TPN bag and paperwork for final pharmacist check.

Automated Compounders

The Nutrimix Macro TPN Compounder pictured below can be programmed to simultaneously pump the four basic ingredients of a TPN (dextrose, water, amino acids, and fat). The Nutrimix Micro TPN Compounder has the capacity to dispense additives, such as electrolytes, into a TPN bag already containing the base components. The pharmacist or the technician needs to program the pumps with the specific gravity and volume needed for each component. Prepare or arrange to observe a TPN preparation using automated compounders.

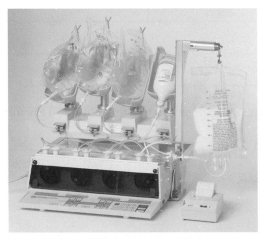

Nutrimix Macro TPN Compounder. (Courtesy of Abbott Hospital Products Division.)

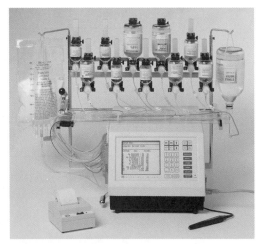

Nutrimix Micro TPN compounder. (Courtesy of Abbott Hospital Products Division.)

Steps:

1. Observe hand-washing and gowning procedures.
2. Observe the set-up of the automated compounder for the base components.
3. Learn the manufacturer protocols for set-up and programming of compounder.
4. Observe the programming of the compounder with the specific gravity and volume of each agent.
5. Some compounders can pump all four components (dextrose, water, amino acids, and fat) at the same time and verify the weights pumped.
6. Observe the set-up of the micro compounder with the additives placed according to manufacturer protocol.
7. Observe programming of compounder with volume and specific gravity of each additive.
8. Compounder will then pump the correct amount of fluid from each vial into the previously mixed base components.
9. If possible, observe daily cleaning and maintenance procedures for the compounders.

▶ Post-Lab Analysis

1. Compare the admixture of total parenteral nutrition formulas using manual procedures and using automated compounders in terms of the following factors:

   Cost_____

   _____

   Accuracy_____

   _____

   Technician time _____

   _____

   Technician training_____

   _____

2. What problem results when fats are added to a three-in-one TPN mixture?

   _____

3. List the information that must be included on the label for a TPN admixture.

_____

_____

_____

_____

4. If a TPN mixture is refrigerated, how soon after the re-warming process begins must the infusion be started?

_____

5. Why is the multivitamin mixture often omitted from the TPN and sent with the bag to be added just before administration?

_____

_____

6. Amelia Ann, the pharmacy technician, is adding trace elements to a TPN bag when she suddenly realizes she is about to sneeze. She manages to turn her head away from the hood and cover her mouth with her gloved hand. What should she do now to prevent contamination of her product?

_____

_____

7. If a LAFW has been turned off, how long must it run before being used to compound sterile preparations?

_____

8. What effect can an increase in room temperature have on IV formulations?

_____

_____

9. How often do refrigerator temperature readings need to be documented when used for storage of IV items?

_____

CHAPTER 19

Chemotherapy Admixture

OBJECTIVES

▸ Use appropriate personal protective equipment when mixing chemotherapeutic agents.

▸ Discuss the added safety precautions required when compounding chemotherapeutic agents.

▸ Demonstrate proper aseptic technique when working in a vertical flow hood.

▸ Demonstrate proper use of a chemo spill kit.

TERMS

Chemotherapeutic agents

PPE

Barrier isolator

MSDS

Antineoplastic drugs

Biological safety cabinet

Vertical flow LAFW

Cytotoxic

Genotoxic

Oncogenic

Mutagenic

Teratogenic

Type B hood

Chemo spill kit

EQUIPMENT

Vertical flow LAFW or simulation

Small-volume parenteral solutions

Syringes and needles

Gown with long sleeves and tight-fitting cuffs

Chemo spill kit

Vials labeled with names of chemo

Hair covers

Shoe covers

Goggles

Gloves

Face masks

Agents that are potentially hazardous to the health play a major role in cancer chemotherapy and the treatment of many other disease conditions. Often they are given by IV infusion and must be prepared in the pharmacy. Technicians must be adequately trained to prepare accurate dosage forms using aseptic technique while adhering to strict safety guidelines to prevent accidental exposure. Each pharmacy stocking hazardous drugs must have written protocols for proper handling and disposal of these drugs as well as written procedures outlining steps to follow in the event of a spill or an exposure incident.

▶ Pre-Lab Questions

1. Briefly describe the difference in a horizontal and a vertical laminar flow hood and why it is important to prepare chemotherapeutic agents in a type B vertical flow laminar hood.

   _____

   _____

   _____

2. List protective apparel that should be worn during chemotherapy IV admixture.

   _____

   _____

   _____

3. Why is double gloving a good safety precaution?

   _____

4. If two pair of gloves are worn, how should they be placed in relationship to the cuff of the gown?

   _____

5. Describe the method for removing and disposing of gloves and disposable gown after the IV is prepared.

   _____

   _____

   _____

6. How many hours a day must a biological safety cabinet run continuously, and how often should it be certified?

_____

_____

7. What size syringe would you choose to draw 5 ml of fluid from a vial? Why?

_____

_____

8. List the contents of a hazardous drug spill kit.

_____

_____

▶ Lab Exercises

Many laboratories may not have access to a biological safety cabinet. In this case, the process may be simulated using a horizontal flow hood with a clear plastic shield at the appropriate height. Drug vials labeled with names of chemotherapeutic agents will also be simulated and not contain hazardous materials. Fill the following orders as if working in a vertical flow hood, being cognizant of the different technique of mixing required and the need to follow all safety precautions required during chemo admixture.

Medication Order 19.1

Date/Time 9/18/05 / 1300   Medication Orders _____

Methotrexate @ 25 g IV in NS 50 ml

Infuse over 15 minutes,
give on days 1 and 8
R. Darren Olson

Patient Information
Henrietta Anderson Hosp ID 65432
Weight: 110, Height: 5'7", 53 yo female

Pharmacy Copy

Steps:

▸ Methotrexate (MTX) is available in the pharmacy in a 10-ml vial with a concentration of 25 mg/ml.

▸ Calculate the number of ml of this MTX solution needed for 1 dose.

_____

▸ This should be double checked and initialed by the pharmacist before mixing.

▸ Follow hand-washing and gowning procedure established by your pharmacy site.

▸ Clean the hood with alcohol.

▸ Gather all materials needed for the compounding.

▸ Arrange materials appropriately so the air flow will not be blocked as you work.

▸ Wipe the top of the MTX vial and the port of the NS bag with alcohol.

▸ Inject an amount of air into the vial equal to $\frac{1}{2}$ to $\frac{3}{4}$ of the amount of methotrexate you will withdraw.

▸ Carefully inject the MTX solution into the port of the NS bag so as not to puncture the bag.

▸ Wipe the port of the IV bag and apply a seal.

▸ Apply IV label and warning label to bag and seal in a bag to prevent leakage.

▸ Follow special chemo protocol for cleanup and disposal of waste.

Medication Order 19.2

Date/Time 9/18/05 / 1300   Medication Orders _____

Fluorouracil 942 mg IV in 50ml NS

Infuse over 10 minutes

Give on days 1 and 8

R. Jason Olson

Patient Information
Henrietta Anderson Hosp ID 65432
Weight: 110, Height: 5'7", 53 yo female

Pharmacy Copy

Steps:

▶ Fluorouracil is available as a prepared solution in a 50-mg/ml concentration.

▶ Calculate the number of ml needed to prepare a dose of 942 mg.

_____

▶ If fluorouracil is available in your pharmacy in 10-ml ampules, how many ampules will you take to the hood? _____

▶ Proceed with proper hand-washing and gowning procedure.

▶ Clean LAFW with alcohol. Be sure hood has been in operation for 24 hours.

▶ Gather all supplies needed for the preparation.

▶ Place the supplies appropriately so as not to interfere with airflow during mixing.

▶ Tap the contents of the ampule until there is no solution left in the top or the neck of the amp. Clean neck of ampule with alcohol.

▶ Attach filter needle to a syringe large enough to hold the amount of solution to be drawn from the syringe.

▶ Draw solution into barrel of syringe and replace filter needle with regular needle.

▶ Expel any air or excess drug (into a sterile vial), and inject the correct amount of drug into NS bag.

▶ Wipe the port of the bag and apply a seal.

▶ Label with IV label, warning label, storage requirements, and expiration date.

▶ Place in sealed bag for final check and transport.

▶ Clean hood of any spills and properly dispose of waste and PPE.

▶ Post-Lab Analysis

1. When filling the MTX order, describe the procedure for maintaining negative pressure in the vial before withdrawing the solution. Why is this important?

_____

_____

_____

_____

2. Check an injectable drug reference book for the appropriate storage and beyond use information to apply to each of these two admixtures.

MTX storage: _____

MTX expiration date: _____

Fluorouracil storage: _____

Fluorouracil expiration date: _____

3. Which reference book did you use for the information in question 2?

   _____

4. There is a loud noise in the pharmacy as you begin to open the fluorouracil ampule, and you accidentally drop the ampule, breaking it and spilling the contents. Describe the procedure you would follow to clean the hood and mix the preparation.

   _____

   _____

   _____

   _____

   _____

5. Why should vials containing cytotoxic materials be stored on shelves that have a guard in front of the shelf?

   _____

6. The unit needing the two IV mixtures is connected to the pharmacy by the pneumatic tube system. The patient has arrived to receive her medications, and they call to have them delivered. Will you send the drugs through the tube or carry it to the room? Why?

   _____

   _____

7. When called to deliver the medication to the patient room "stat," you leave the hood to be cleaned after you return. Will you need to put on any protective equipment just to clean the hood? If so, what would you need?

   _____

   _____

   _____

8. Should the fan on the hood be turned on or off during the cleaning process?

   _____

9. The technician who is scheduled to mix chemotherapy medications confides in you that she thinks she may be pregnant. Would this be a concern? What action would you take?

_____

_____

10. While cleaning the hood, the outside glove on your left hand snags and is torn. What would you do?

_____

_____

Supplemental Prescriptions and Medication Orders

The following prescriptions will provide practice in completing the prescription-filling process from beginning to end. After completing the first three chapters, these prescriptions should each be accepted from a "patient" with appropriate information-gathering skills. They should then be entered into the pharmacy software and filled, and appropriate labels and auxiliary labels should be applied. The prescription and paperwork should then be left in the designated area for a final check by the instructor. Refer to the step-by-step processes learned in the first three chapters to complete this exercise. Blanks are provided alongside each prescription so that the student can take notes.

Two supplemental medication orders are also included after the prescriptions.

PRESCRIPTION 1

Dr. Alfred Sauls
151212 S. High Rd., Chicago, IL 23875
954-555-1300

Name: Alan Johnson   92 Ibis Lane

RX: lanoxin 0.25

Disp: # 100

Sig: 1 tablet po qd

Dr. Alfred Sauls

Dispense as written   May substitute

_____

_____

_____

_____

_____

PRESCRIPTION 2

Dr. Alfred Sauls
151212 S. High Rd., Chicago, IL 23875
954-555-1300

Name: Jonathan Swanson   42 Spring St.

RX: Coumadin 5.0 mg
Sig: 1 tablet M-F
       1/2 tablet Sat-Sun
Disp: # 45

Dr. Alfred Sauls

Dispense as written   May substitute

_____

_____

_____

_____

PRESCRIPTION 3

Dr. Martin Schwartz
98 North Ridge, New York, NY 88364
813-455-7554

Name: Mary Green   81 SW 6th St.

RX: Coumadin 5 mg

Disp: #30

Sig: i po daily

☐ Label

Refill _____ times (PRN)   NR

Dr. Martin Schwartz

Dispense as written   May substitute

_____

_____

_____

_____

PRESCRIPTION 4

Dr. Calvin Robins
7823 Tea Rose Trail, Miami, FL 44718
463-555-8000

Name: Jack Davis   500 SE 2 St.

RX:

Disp: #50

_____   Dr. Calvin Robins
Dispense as written   May substitute

PRESCRIPTION 5

Dr. Doug Griffin
7611 147th Terrace, Monterey, CA 38411
705-555-6644

Name: Andrea Kelly   474 Hurricane Alley

RX: Prilosec

Disp: # XXX

Sig: one daily

_____   Dr. Doug Griffin
Dispense as written   May substitute

PRESCRIPTION 6

Dr. Debra Lawson
888 NW 27th Ave., Miami, FL 98885
247-555-6613

Name: Virginia Millhouse   678 Apple St.

RX: Amoxicillin Cap.
250

Disp:

Sig: i 3 Times daily
as needed for
bladder urinary for 3 days
Qty. # 30

Refill ___1___ times

_____   Dr. Debra Lawson
Dispense as written   May substitute

PRESCRIPTION 7

Dr. Angelina Teveso
8809 21st Ave., Brooklyn, NY 88364
812-444-2929

Name: Thelma Harris   7100 New Utrecht Ave.

RX: _Restail 15 y_

Disp: _# 30_

Sig: _Tus PRN_

Refill ___I___ times   PRN   NR

Dr. A. Teveso

_____   _____
Dispense as written   May substitute

PRESCRIPTION 8

Dr. Lawrence Krinsky
13 North Ridge, New York, NY 88364
813-555-1313

Name: Harold Baker   99 West St.

RX: _Restoril 15_

Disp: _Tro tts PRN_

Sig: _# 30_

Dr. Lawrence Krinsky

_____   _____
Dispense as written   May substitute

PRESCRIPTION 9

Dr. Howard Isaacs
1115 Turnaround Lane, Detroit, MI 64789
343-555-7000

Name: Barbara Erickson   854 Green St.

RX: _Oxycodone c APAP_

Disp: _# 60_

Sig: _T PC q6° PRN_

Dr. Howard Isaacs

_____   _____
Dispense as written   May substitute

PRESCRIPTION 10

Dr. Donna Johns
7000 SW 1st Ave., Santa Fe, NM 54545
766-555-9097

Name: James Wilson   53 Iris Blvd.

RX:

Dr. Donna Johns

Dispense as written   May substitute

PRESCRIPTION 11

Dr. Agnes Cooper
55 North Ridge, New York, NY 88364
813-555-7777

Name: Dennis Williams   33 Paine

RX:

Disp:

Sig:

Dr. Agnes Cooper

Dispense as written   May substitute

PRESCRIPTION 12

Dr. Gaudy Sotolongo
55 North Ridge, New York, NY 88364
813-555-7557

Name: David Brushwood   88 SW 6th St.

RX:

Disp:

Sig:

Label
Refill _____ times   PRN   NR

Dr. Gaudy Sotolongo

Dispense as written   May substitute

PRESCRIPTION 13

Dr. Barry Weiss
901 Sheridan St., Austin, TX 90902
874-555-9000

Name: Bob Thomas   894 West Rd.

RX: Casix 40mg

Disp: Tabs Ti po q AM

Sig: #60

_____   _Dr. Barry Weiss_
Dispense as written   May substitute

PRESCRIPTION 14

Dr. Doug Griffin
7611 147th Terrace, Monterey, CA 38411
705-555-6644

Name: Lisa Adams   53 Iris Blvd.

RX:

Disp: Lasix 40mg #100
Sig: tab T bid

_____   _Dr. Doug Griffin_
Dispense as written   May substitute

PRESCRIPTION 15

Dr. Barry Weiss
901 Sheridan St., Austin, TX 90902
874-555-1300

Name: Katherine Smith   498 E 11th St.

RX: Lasix 40mg

Disp: #30

Sig T q am

_____   _Dr. Barry Weiss_
Dispense as written   May substitute

PRESCRIPTION 16

Dr. Erin Thomas
988 North Ridge, New York, NY 88364
813-555-7554

Name: Marjorie Jones   154 Oriole Ave.

RX: Lipitor 10 mg

Disp: #60

Sig: i TiD Daily

Dr. Erin Thomas

_____   _____
Dispense as written   May substitute

PRESCRIPTION 17

Dr. Doug Griffin
7611 147th Terrace, Monterey, CA 38411
705-555-6644

Name: Mathew Johnson   71 Capitol Ave.

RX: Amoxil

Disp: 250mg/T5
100 5

Sig: 3/4 tsp po. ~1/0
X 10 DAys

Dr. Doug Griffin

_____   _____
Dispense as written   May substitute

PRESCRIPTION 18

Dr. Eleanor Salerno
2799 Victory Place, East Brunswick, NJ 33838
400-555-3344

Name: Monrose Gifford   23 NW 4th Ct.

RX: Humulin NPH   1bottle
25U each morning
20U each evening

Regular Humulin Insulin   1bottle
SSI - use per scale
given

Dr. E. Salerno

_____   _____
Dispense as written   May substitute

MEDICATION ORDER 1

Date/Time	Orders	Progress Notes

3/9/01 1300	Admit: GMF
	Dx: pyelonephritis
	    HTN
	    Type 2 DM
	    hyperlipidemia
	Condition: good
	VS: q shift
	Activity: up ad lib
	Nursing: I & O's, Accuchecks AC+HS
	Diet: ADA 2000 calorie
	Allergies: Sulfa
	Meds: Rocephin 1gm IV q24°
	    Accupril 20mg p.o. qd
	    glucophage 500mg p.o. BID
	    Lipitor 40mg p.o. qd
	    Demerol 50mg IM q4-6° PRN pain
	    Pyridium 200mg p.o. TID x 2 days
	    Tylenol 500mg p.o. BID PRN fever
	    Restoril 15mg p.o. qHS PRN insomnia
	    Compazine 25mg p.o. q8° PRN nausea
	Labs:
	    CBC, Chem 22, KUB
	    Renal Ultrasound
		54 y/o ♀ c̄ h/o HTN, DM, ↑lipids
		presents c̄ 2 days of worsening
		Ⓛ side low back pain, dysuria
		and fever. She does have a
		h/o frequent UTI's; last one
		several months ago. She
		states she also has lower abd
		pain and some nausea ō emesis.
		pt notes blood in urine
		PMHx: HTN, DM, ↑lipids
		PSHx: hysterectomy
		FHx: CAD, HTN, CVA
		SocHx: Divorced - receptionist
		    ⊕ Tob lppd soc ETOH ō illicits
		All: Sulfa meds: Accupril 20 qd
		                    glucophage 500 BID
		                    Lipitor 40 qd
		Ⓖ A/O x 3 NAD
		    VSS T~100°
		CV - RRR Lungs - CTA
		Abd - soft tender suprapubic +BS
		    ⊕ CVAT
		Ext - ō CCE
		A/P 1) pyelonephritis 2) DM 3) HTN
		    4) ↑lipids
		Admit, IV antibx, pain control
		IVF — continue current meds

PATIENT INFORMATION

Jane Doe 54 y/o
2-23-50

MEDICAL ORDERS AND PROGRESS NOTES

EL-FR-NR-1001-1101

CHART COPY

MEDICATION ORDER 2

Date/Time	Orders	Progress Notes

2/23/04 800	Admit – Tele unit
	Dx's: Chest Pain R/o MI
	HTN
	Condition: guarded
	V.S. q2° NKDA
	Activity: Bedrest
	Nursing – guiac stools
	 īs CP → obtain EKG
	Diet: cardiac Diet 2gm Nā
	IVNS @ 80cc/hr° cate
	O₂ NC 2L/min
	ASA 325mg p.o. qd
	SL NTG 0.4mg SL q5min
	Till painfree
	Norvasc 5mg p.o. qd
	Tylenol 650mg p.o. q6°/PRN
	Ativan 2mg p.o. q8°/PRN: Anxiety
	Mylanta 30cc p.o. q10/PRN dyspepsia
	Labs: CXR PA/LAT
	EKG
	Serial cardiac enzymes
	CBC, chem 22
	PT/INR/PTT
	Schedule cardiac stress
	Test in AM
	MS 2-4mg IV q4-6°/PRN pain
		64 y/o ♂ c̄ 4/o HTN presents
		Today p̄ having SSCP
		p̄ shoveling snow from
		driveway. CP resolved
		p̄ he sat down to rest
		Pt denies Nausea/Diaphoresis
		or radiation of pain
		to arm.
		PmHx: HTN PSHx: Lasix
		NKDA meds Norvasc 5gqd
		Soc Retired widow Tob ⊘ illicit
		FHx: noncontributory BETOH
		○ gen A/O NAD
		  VSS EKG NSR ⊘ ST/TWAV D's
		
		CV – RRR s̄ m/R/G
		Lungs – CTA ⊘ R/B/W
		Abd – soft NT/ND ⊕ BS
		Ext – ⊘ CCE
		
		A/P 1) CP R/o MI
		  2) HTN
		
		Admit Tele – serial enzymes
		Labs, stress Test in AM

MEDICAL ORDERS AND PROGRESS NOTES

EL-FR-NR-1001-1101

PATIENT INFORMATION

Joe Doe 64 y/o
9-28-40

CHART COPY